Do It Right

The **75** Best Body-Sculpting Exercises for Women

From the Editors of

SHAPE

ACKNOWLEDGEMENTS

This special publication is based on articles written by Mark Cibrario, C.S.C.S., Karen Clippinger, M.S.P.E., Deborah Ellison, P.T., Dawn Norman, M.S., A.T.C., and Linda Shelton for SHAPE magazine. Photography by James Allen, Larry Bartholomew, Adam Brown, Don Flood, Shannon Greer, Dominick Guillemot, John McKee, Willie Maldonado and Mike Russ. Illustrations by Karen Kuchar. Project Editor is Jeanine Detz. Project and cover design by Kimberly Richey. SHAPE Fitness Director is Linda Shelton. SHAPE Director of Photography is Melissa O'Brien. SHAPE Assistant Photo Editor is Arlyn Petalver. Production Manager is Renee Thompson. Director of Rights and Permissions is Fiona Maynard. SHAPE Editor in Chief is Anne M. Russell. EVP, Editorial Director, Active Lifestyle Group, is Barbara Harris. EVP, Chief Editorial Director is Bonnie Fuller. Founding Chairman is Joe Weider.
Chairman, President, CEO is David Pecker.

Special thanks to our reader models: Sarah Gorgita, Irene Goryn, Kim Hicks, Brooke Hobbs, Billie Hoekstra, Kristin Isler, Shachella James, Katie Knopp, Andrea Naud, Jamie Oldfield, Arlyn Petalver, Lindsay Robinson, Karen Salt, Darlene Salvador, Amie Stoeber, Leah Tribble, Melinda Vassberg and Maggie Welter.

CONTENTS

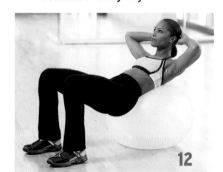

12

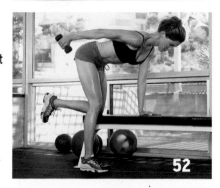

52

INTRODUCTION

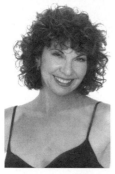

Seeing positive results from your training gives you a fabulous boost of confidence and motivates you to stay on the fitness path.

If your body isn't as lean or toned as you'd like, or your muscles are slow in responding to your current program, you may be committing some fundamental training blunders.

The good news is, some of the biggest training errors can be fixed with the smallest of solutions – a slight change in posture, a nominal increase in the weight of a dumbbell, a shift in arm position or leg position. An incremental change in your form can have a huge impact on how your body responds.

With time a valuable commodity, you want to get the best return for the time you invest in your workouts. *Do It Right* is a step-by-step guide designed to teach you how to maximize exercise benefits and to get better results from your fitness program than ever before. Rather than training harder, the key is training smarter! Proper form is everything. Stay focused and mindful of good posture, balance and control each time you work out. This is the smart way to build a solid fitness foundation as well as to take your training to the next level.

Do It Right is a compilation of exercises from one of SHAPE's most popular columns. It offers in-depth information on 75 popular exercises targeted to the body parts women want to sculpt the most: abs, arms, back, butt, chest, hips and thighs, and shoulders. Each exercise includes "The Right Way" (the correct technique), "The Payoff" (benefits), "Muscles Worked," "Workout Guidelines" (how many sets, reps and weight suggestions), "Expert Advice" and "Mistakes to Avoid." There's also a section with 10 must-do stretches to keep your muscles flexible for strength training.

HOW TO USE THIS BOOK

What exercises should you choose? What order should you do them in? How much weight should you lift?

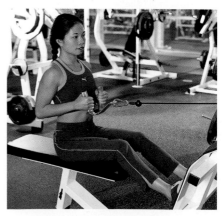

How many reps and sets should you do? Planning a solid strength-training program involves asking these important questions because the answers ensure that your program is well-rounded, complete and, most important, supports your goals. Once you establish your starting level, there are plenty of exercises to choose from to give you a challenging yet manageable workout.

Each chapter is organized according to difficulty: beginning, intermediate and advanced. Even if you've been training a while, start with novice-level exercises to reteach your body the biomechanics of each movement. As you progress, the beginning exercises can be cycled in to vary your training program.

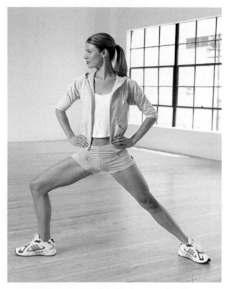

TO BEGIN, FOLLOW THESE 3 EASY STEPS:
1. READY: Choose your fitness level.
- If you've been sedentary or have been training for three months or less, start with beginner exercises.
- If you've been consistently training a minimum of twice a week for three months or more, include both beginner and intermediate exercises in your program.
- If you've been training 2-3 times a week for six months or more, consider yourself advanced and use any of the exercises in your program. For more of a challenge, see the suggestions listed in "Workout Guidelines" to progress.
2. SET: Determine your program

goal, time constraints, and where you'll train.
- What do you want to accomplish?
- Do you want to build strength, get toned, train for a sport?
- How much time can you commit to your program each week?
- Do you train at home, at a gym, or both?

3. GO: Create your personal training program.
Use the following recommendations to plan your program:
Number of Training Days Strength training your total body 2-3 times per week on nonconsecutive days is sufficient for most women. (Advanced training, such as split routines working one to three body parts a day, usually requires 4-6 days per week.)
Rest Take one to two days off between workouts, depending on your workout intensity.
Number of Exercises: To maintain

posture, muscle balance, symmetry and strength, include at least one exercise for every major muscle group, based on your fitness level. A complete strength-training program works all the major muscles, not necessarily in the same workout, but all should be worked twice weekly on nonconsecutive days.

Exercise Selection Include both single- and multijoint exercises in your program. A single-joint exercise is isolation training; you work only one joint at a time. Examples of these exercises include the biceps curl, lateral raise and prone hamstring curl. Multijoint training works many muscles at once. The squat, lunge and overhead press are all multijoint movements.

Exercise Progression Choose exercises that are safe for you. That means you are able to complete them using good form. If you're a beginner, stick with the minimum recommendations and increase your workout gradually, when the workload is no longer challenging.

Exercise Order In general, work your largest muscles first — say, your legs or back — especially if you're lifting heavy weights.

Amount of Weight Work with as heavy a weight as you can, using good form to complete all recommended reps and sets.

Variety To keep muscles responding and to avoid an exercise plateau, change your exercises regularly.

Our book arms you with enough training information to get started and stay motivated. Regardless of your level or your knowledge about training, you'll find this to be more than just another strength-training book. *Do It Right* is a comprehensive reference guide that can get you amazing results!

Linda Shelton

Linda Shelton
SHAPE Fitness Director

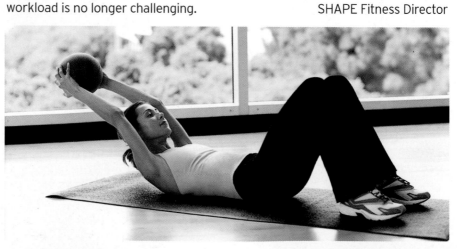

ABDOMINAL EXERCISES

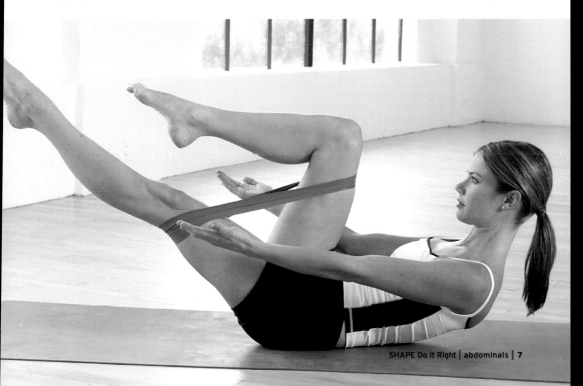

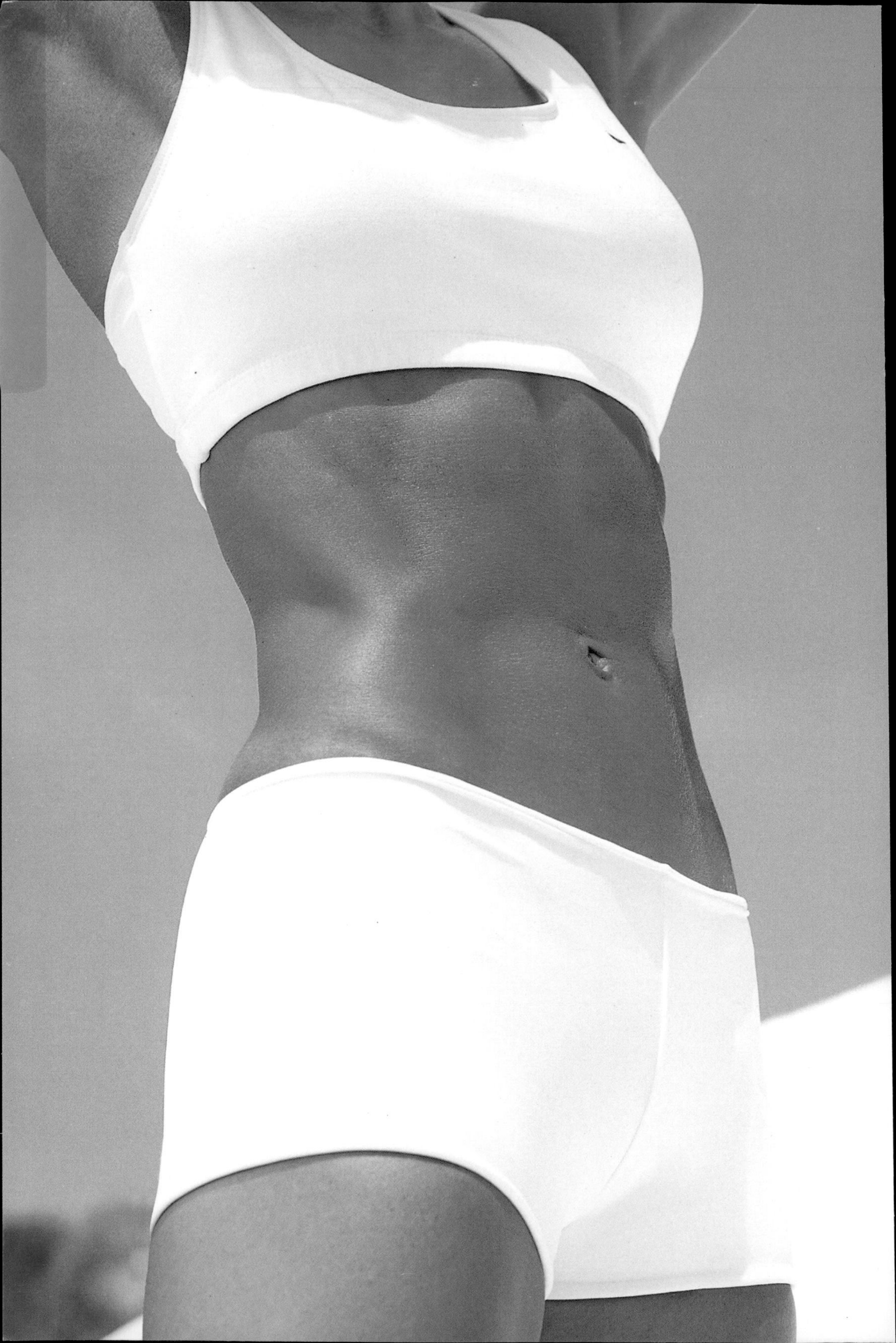

ABDOMINALS

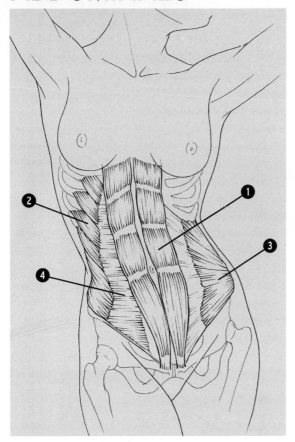

MUSCLES
1. rectus abdominis
2. external obliques
3. internal obliques
4. transverse abdominis

The abdominals are comprised of four muscle groups: rectus abdominis, external obliques, internal obliques and transverse abdominis. The rectus abdominis runs from the top of the pubic bone to the sternum and flexes the torso. Attached to the connective tissue of the rectus abdominis are the external obliques, running diagonally downward from the lower ribs to the mid-portion of the upper pelvis bone. The internal obliques run diagonally upward from the pelvis to the lower ribs. Both oblique groups work with the rectus abdominis to flex, unilaterally rotate and laterally flex the torso. The transverse abdominis, a deep muscle running horizontally from back to front, contracts when the others are working but can't be isolated. The abdominals work both as primary movers and stabilizers of the spine.

You'll stand taller by putting a new angle on your abdominal work.

THE RIGHT WAY

➤ Lie on your side, knees bent at a 45-degree angle, feet relaxed and crossed at the ankles. Rock your body back as a unit until your knees lift 8 inches off floor.

➤ With fingertips lightly at the back of your head, slowly curl up on a diagonal. Focus on lifting the torso with the abdominal muscles, sequentially lifting your head, shoulders and torso.

➤ Bring lower ribs toward the top of hip and pull the whole abdominal wall inward. Keep elbows back; don't pull on neck.

➤ Bring arms forward and curl up slightly higher, still keeping the side of the pelvis on the floor. Then, slowly bring hands to the back of your head without letting torso drop.

➤ Hold for 4 counts; slowly lower torso, shoulders, then head to starting position.

➤ Throughout the exercise, focus on keeping the torso slightly rounded forward as you twist up.

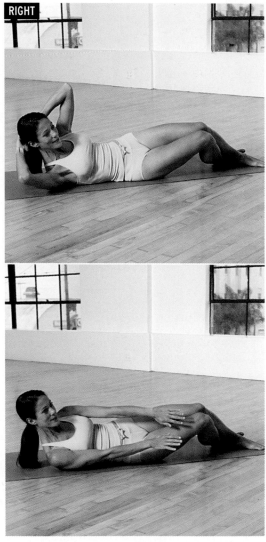

RIGHT

MUSCLES WORKED
internal obliques, external obliques, rectus abdominis, transverse abdominis

ABS SIDE-UP

THE PAYOFF

You know your muscles need variety: You've mixed up your cardio stints, but you probably still end each session with a steady diet of abdominal crunches. It's time to shake up your ab routine, too. This move challenges the side abdominal muscles – the obliques – regardless of your fitness level. The side-up tones up these muscles, helping to improve your posture and prevent lower-back injury.

WORKOUT GUIDELINES

Do 1 set of 6 reps per side, working up to 12 reps. Rest 45 to 60 seconds between sides, then repeat the sequence for 1 more set. When you can do 2 sets of 12 with correct form, progress by holding a 1 to 3 pound weight in each hand.

EXPERT ADVICE

"Focus on keeping the torso slightly rounded forward as you twist up," says Karen Clippinger, M.S.P.E., a Los Angeles-based kinesiologist and instructor at UCLA. "This helps to engage the abdominals throughout the entire exercise."

This move effectively challenges the side abdominal muscles – the obliques – regardless of your fitness level.

MISTAKES TO AVOID

➤ **Don't** lead with your chin, pull on your neck or jam your chin into your neck; this can cause cervical neck strain.

➤ **Don't** use speed or momentum to curl up; you'll take the emphasis off your abdominals and put stress on your lower back.

➤ **Don't** over-rotate and roll to one side as you lift. This decreases exercise efficiency and pulls on your back muscles.

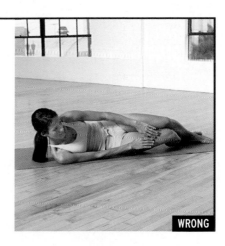

WRONG

A better way to crunch for a sleeker, sexier midsection.

abdominals

THE RIGHT WAY

➤ Sit upright on a stability ball, knees bent at 90 degrees, thighs about parallel to floor, feet flat.

➤ Walk both feet forward so ball rolls up spine until it's under your mid- to lower back. Your torso should be just about parallel to the floor (or upper back can be slightly lower; see "Expert Advice.")

➤ Keeping your feet flat, about hip-width apart, ankles directly in line with knees, place fingertips behind head, unclasped, squeezing shoulder blades together and tightening buttocks to stabilize position.

➤ Contract abdominals as you exhale, pulling lower rib cage downward and curling torso up and in toward hips, lower back pressing firmly against ball.

➤ Continue curling until abdominals reach full contraction (just before lower back begins to release from ball), then slowly return to start position.

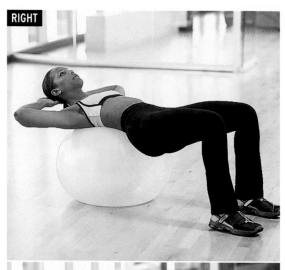

RIGHT

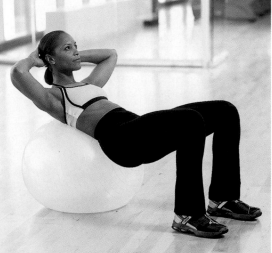

MUSCLES WORKED
rectus abdominis, external obliques, internal obliques, transverse abdominis

STABILITY-BALL CRUNCH

THE PAYOFF

The standard crunch is enhanced on a stability ball because your abs, particularly the oblique muscles, are forced to work harder as you maintain your balance. Your body is also better cushioned than on the floor; plus you achieve a greater range of motion.

WORKOUT GUIDELINES

Use a 55- or 65-centimeter ball, depending upon your height; your thighs should be parallel to the floor when sitting upright on the ball. Do 1-2 sets of 15 reps, resting 1-2 minutes between sets. To progress, work up to 25 reps per set. For a greater challenge: Extend arms above head; or walk feet forward and balance on your heels.

EXPERT ADVICE

"To really work ab muscles, extend your spine over the ball, lowering trunk slightly below parallel position by dropping shoulders and arms below top of ball," says Douglas Brooks, M.S., a specialist in exercise physiology and a personal trainer in Northern California. "This increases the range of motion and gives you better command of your abdominal muscles."

The standard crunch is enhanced on a stability ball because your abs work harder as you maintain your balance.

MISTAKES TO AVOID

➤ **Don't** release your abs as you return to the start position; you may force your back to hyperextend, placing unnecessary stress on surrounding ligaments and discs.
➤ **Don't** tilt head forward or drop head back; this may strain the neck.
➤ **Don't** rock and roll up to a seated position; this will cause the ball to move forward and will make the exercise less efficient.

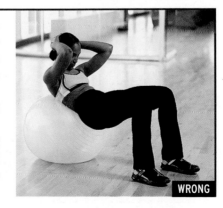

WRONG

A simple way to stronger abs, better posture and a pain-free back.

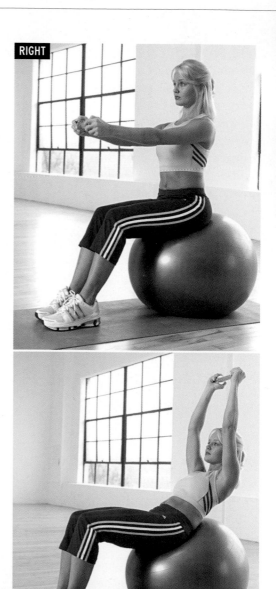

RIGHT

abdominals

THE RIGHT WAY

➤ Sit erect on a stability ball, knees bent, feet flat on floor. Hold a dumbbell with one hand on either end, arms extended in front of you at chest height.

➤ Squeeze shoulder blades down and together, then contract abdominal muscles to tilt pelvis to stabilize position, continuing to use your abs to roll backward onto the ball until back is firmly on the ball from tailbone to lower back. Torso is at a 45-degree angle to the floor.

➤ With abdominals firmly contracted and torso stabilized, extend arms overhead until they're slightly in front of ears.

➤ Hold for 4 counts, then lower dumbbell and repeat the overhead lift, maintaining position. Complete reps, then curl your upper ribs toward your pelvis as you slowly return torso to start position.

MUSCLES WORKED
rectus abdominis, external obliques, internal obliques, transverse abdominis

BALL CURL-DOWN

THE PAYOFF

By starting upright, as you do with the ball curl-down, you work through a larger range of motion and generate greater force than you would by lying on the floor. You also use your abs in conjunction with other torso muscles to keep the ball stable and your body balanced on top.

WORKOUT GUIDELINES

Do 1 to 3 sets of 6 to 12 reps, rolling up to start position and resting 60 seconds between sets. When you can do 3 sets of 12 reps, progress by lowering torso to a more parallel position with the floor. Use a 5- to 8-pound dumbbell.

EXPERT ADVICE

"To work your abs rather than the hip flexors, focus on keeping your torso as rounded as possible, pelvis tilted and lower ribs pulled down and toward your spine," says Karen Clippinger, M.S.P.E., Los Angeles-based kinesiologist and instructor at UCLA. "Keeping your spine flat instead of curved decreases the amount of abdominal involvement and it may also strain your back."

By starting upright, you generate greater force than you would by lying on the floor.

MISTAKES TO AVOID

➤ **Don't** drop your torso lower than parallel to the floor; this places excess strain on your back.
➤ **Don't** lower your arms so far behind your head that it causes your back to arch and your ribs to pop out.
➤ **Don't** keep your spine straight as you lower. You'll put stress on your lower back.

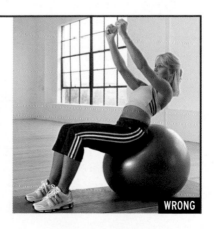

WRONG

Want stronger abs in less time? Try the multi-arc curl-up.

abdominals

THE RIGHT WAY

➤ Lie on your back, knees bent, feet a comfortable distance from your buttocks. Place your fingertips lightly on your head, elbows out.

➤ Slowly curl up diagonally toward your right thigh, first lifting your head, then your neck and shoulder blades. Think about pulling the lower ribs toward the navel and keeping the torso as rounded as possible. Keep the abdominals pulled firmly toward the spine throughout the curl.

➤ Reach forward to grasp the outside of your right thigh with both hands, pulling the torso slightly higher. Let go of your thigh and hold the position for four counts, then slowly put your hands back on your head. Slowly lower your torso to the floor. Repeat.

MUSCLES WORKED
rectus abdominis, external and internal obliques, transverse abdominis

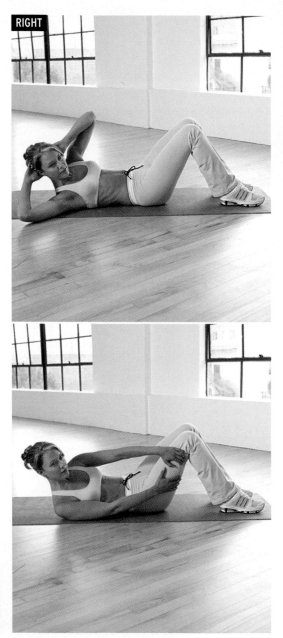

RIGHT

MULTI-ARC CURL-UP

THE PAYOFF

Who wouldn't want a stronger, flatter abdomen? Not many of us, if the popularity of abdominal training is any indicator. In addition to looking great, strong abdominals can help improve your posture and prevent low-back injury. To reap more benefits from ab training in less time, work the multi-arc curl-up into your training program. The change of arm position in this exercise offers more challenge in terms of resistance and range of motion.

WORKOUT GUIDELINES

Do 2 sets of 8 to 12 reps on each side (1 set equals reps on both sides); rest 1 minute between sides. To progress, do the same move with feet placed farther away from your hips on the floor. No weight required.

EXPERT ADVICE

"Think about pulling the lower ribs toward the navel and keeping the torso as rounded as possible," says Karen Clippinger, Los Angeles-based kinesiologist and instructor at UCLA. "Focus on keeping the abdominals pulled in firmly toward the spine throughout the entire movement."

The change of arm position in this exercise offers more challenge in terms of resistance and range of motion.

MISTAKES TO AVOID

➤ **Don't** curl up too quickly or use momentum; this places stress on the back, particularly when you're working on a diagonal.

➤ **Don't** lift up so high that your back comes up off the floor. This forces you to rely on the hip flexors to sustain the position, and may add extra stress to your lower back.

➤ **Don't** lift with a straight back as this strains the lower back muscles and ligaments.

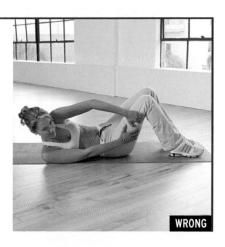

WRONG

Crunched for time? Battle the bulge with this supereffective ab move.

abdominals

THE RIGHT WAY

➤ Lie on your back, bend your knees, raising them so they're in line with your hips, calves parallel to floor. Place thumbs behind ears, fingertips touching behind head.

➤ Contract your abs, bringing your lower ribs and hips together to stabilize the pelvis.

➤ Keeping left knee bent and stable, extend right leg to a 45-degree angle at the hip while using abs to rotate and raise the right shoulder toward the left knee, keeping elbows open as you lift head, neck and shoulder blades off the floor.

➤ Return upper torso to the floor as you bend right knee back to start position, then repeat move on other side to complete 1 rep.

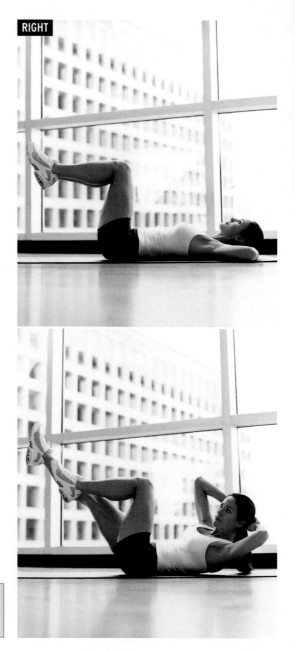

RIGHT

MUSCLES WORKED
rectus abdominis, external obliques,
internal obliques, transverse abdominis

BICYCLES

THE PAYOFF
Scientifically proven to be one of the most effective abdominal exercises, this crunch helps you sculpt your entire torso, all the way down to your deepest abdominal layer. By contracting and strengthening all your abdominal muscles at once, particularly the oblique muscles on the sides of your torso, you'll get a flatter belly and make "love handles" less likely.

WORKOUT GUIDELINES
Perform 2–3 sets of 10–15 reps (1 rep equals both sides). Rest for 45–60 seconds after each set.

When 15 reps are no longer challenging, progress to 20 reps per set.

EXPERT ADVICE
"Rotate your entire upper torso toward the stable knee as you extend the other leg," says Evanston, Ill., strength and conditioning specialist CC Cunningham, M.S., a spokeswoman for the American Council on Exercise. "This will help you focus your efforts on the down stroke of the movement, rather than on the knee pulled in toward your chest, placing maximum tension on your abs."

By contracting and strengthening all your abdominal muscles at once, you'll get a flatter belly.

MISTAKES TO AVOID

➤ **Don't** rock your hips from side to side as you change legs; this prevents your abs from working to stabilize you.
➤ **Don't** wrap your arms around your head or clasp your hands; this can strain your neck and shoulders.
➤ **Don't** "cycle" your legs as fast as you can; this causes you to use momentum rather than slow, controlled movements and prevents the abs from working hard.

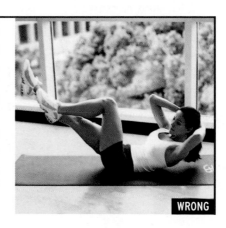

WRONG

Add resistance to your crunches for an even firmer, stronger midsection.

THE RIGHT WAY

➤ Lie on your back with knees bent, and feet flat on the floor, slightly separated.

➤ Holding a medicine ball with both hands, lift your arms above your head, arms slightly bent and in line with your ears.

➤ Contract your abdominals to bring your spine to a neutral position, buttocks relaxed.

➤ Maintain arm position as you curl your torso upward, moving smoothly as one unit, flexing only from the spine and bringing ribs and hips toward each other to lift shoulder blades off the floor.

➤ Pause at the top, then lower to starting position.

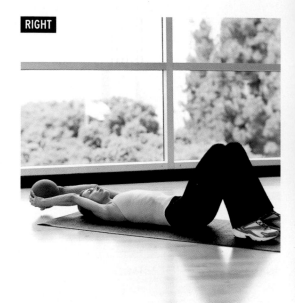

RIGHT

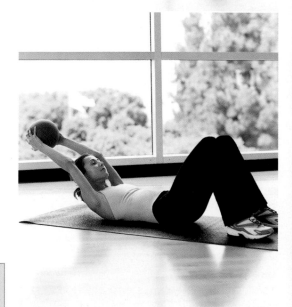

MUSCLES WORKED
rectus abdominis, external obliques, internal obliques, transverse abdominis

MEDICINE-BALL OVERHEAD CRUNCH

THE PAYOFF

Performing your crunches with a medicine ball makes training your abdominals more efficient, challenging and effective, as the added weight helps to fatigue your muscles in fewer reps. You'll work your entire midsection evenly, yielding flatter, firmer abs in less time.

WORKOUT GUIDELINES

Use a 2- to 6-pound medicine ball, making sure not to impede your form with too much weight. Begin with 2 sets of 10-15 reps, resting 1 minute between sets. To progress, add a third set.

EXPERT ADVICE

"Keep your arms extended and motionless by your ears as you lift your torso upward," says Lafayette, La.-based Mike Morris, NASM-certified personal trainer and president of Resist-A-Ball Inc. "This maximizes the strengthening effect on the abs and ensures that you're not using momentum to 'throw' the ball over your head as you execute the crunch."

Doing your crunches with a medicine ball makes training your abdominals more challenging and effective.

MISTAKES TO AVOID

➤ **Don't** use a ball so heavy that you don't have a full range of motion; this will stress the neck and shoulders.

➤ **Don't** arch your back as you return to the starting position, lifting arms overhead; this can place pressure on the discs in the lower back.

➤ **Don't** jerk your body into position as you lift your upper torso; this will place stress on the spine and neck.

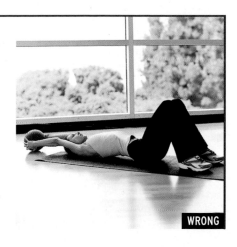

WRONG

Get amazing abs, arms and shoulders with one move.

THE RIGHT WAY

➤ Begin on your hands and knees, with your wrists directly under your shoulders. Your arms should be straight, your fingers pointing straight ahead and your knees lined up directly under each hip.

➤ Contract your abdominal muscles, pulling your navel toward your spine so your body forms a straight line from your head to your hips. Find your center of balance so your arms and thighs are perfectly vertical and parallel to each other.

➤ Slightly raise one of your legs and extend it behind you. Place the ball of that foot on the floor. Then extend the other leg behind you and place the ball of that foot on floor, maintaining your torso position.

➤ As you balance on your hands and the balls of your feet, your body should be in the plank pose, forming a straight line from your head to your heels.

➤ Be sure to keep your buttocks contracted and your leg and abdominal muscles tight in order to maintain the position. Hold this pose for 30 seconds.

RIGHT

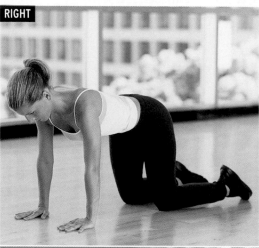

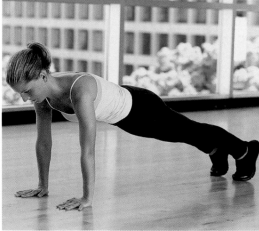

MUSCLES WORKED
rectus abdominis, external obliques, internal obliques, transverse abdominis, triceps, biceps, deltoids

PLANK

THE PAYOFF
More than just a yoga pose or preparation for a push-up, this ultra-effective move tightens and tones the abdominal muscles, gives your arms and shoulders definition and strengthens your back and leg muscles. Having a sleeker, stronger core of muscles will make you look and feel better in everything you do.

WORKOUT GUIDELINES
Begin by holding your body in the plank position for 30 seconds. As you progress, strive to hold it for 45-60 seconds if possible. To progress, alternately lift one leg.

EXPERT ADVICE
"To ensure that you use correct alignment, look straight down at your arms and line your elbow creases up with the tops of your wrists," says Leigh Crews, National Academy of Sports Medicine and Cooper Institute-certified trainer and owner of Dynalife Fitness Inc. in Rome, Ga. "This helps distribute your weight equally between arms and legs and maintain a straight line from head to heels."

> More than just a yoga pose or preparation for a push-up, this move tones the abdominal muscles.

MISTAKES TO AVOID

➤ **Don't** let your belly sag toward the floor; doing so will place stress on your lower back that could lead to injury.

➤ **Don't** let your head drop or your shoulders hunch up toward your ears; if you do this, your arms, shoulders, back and abdominal muscles will be doing less of the work.

➤ **Don't** let your hips lift up into a "V" position; this will give you less core strength.

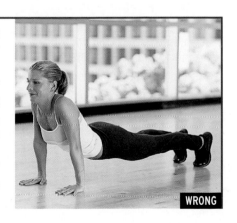

WRONG

Not just a belly buster, this move strengthens your entire core.

THE RIGHT WAY

➤ Lie on your back, legs bent, hands holding legs behind thighs.

➤ Inhale, then exhale, drawing navel in and back toward spine to draw in abs. Move knees out until they're directly above hips; shins parallel to floor.

➤ Look toward your navel; peel head and shoulders off the floor until shoulder blades are off the mat. Straighten arms beside body, palms down, hovering above mat. (If you feel neck strain, put hands behind head.)

➤ Keeping arms straight, extend legs at a 45-degree angle to the floor, keeping knees and ankles together and pointing toes.

➤ Pump arms downward from shoulders, inhaling deeply for five counts, then exhaling for five counts, continuing to draw abs inward.

➤ Maintain position for as many sets as you can handle without straining neck, then lower to starting position.

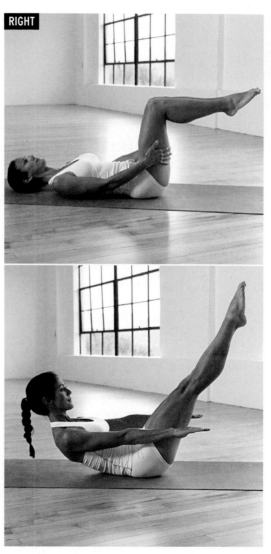

RIGHT

MUSCLES WORKED
rectus abdominis, internal obliques, external obliques, transverse abdominis

PILATES HUNDRED

THE PAYOFF

The Pilates Hundred is the first move in the original series of Pilates mat exercises. It is a core strengthening exercise, as opposed to just an abdominal crunch. By maintaining and holding a steady position, you force your abdominal and back muscles to work together, helping you build muscle endurance, tightening your midsection, improving posture and strengthening your upper back stabilizer muscles.

WORKOUT GUIDELINES

Begin with 5 sets of the exercise (inhale/exhale every 5 breaths), and progress up to 100, which is 10 sets of the breath. If necessary, keep knees bent in set-up position until you're strong enough to maintain alignment with legs extended.

EXPERT ADVICE

"Don't let your abdominals poke out like a loaf of bread," says Elizabeth Larkam, M.A., a Pilates specialist and Reebok Trainer from Marin County, Calif. "Instead, imagine 'zipping' up your abs as if you were putting on a tight pair of jeans."

The Pilates Hundred tightens your midsection, improves posture and helps prevent lower-back pain.

MISTAKES TO AVOID

➤ **Don't** drop your head back or raise it too far; this places strain on your neck muscles.

➤ **Don't** lower your legs below 45 degrees; You can stress your lower back and compromise using your abdominals.

➤ **Don't** pump your arms so vigorously that it becomes an arm exercise; use your abs.

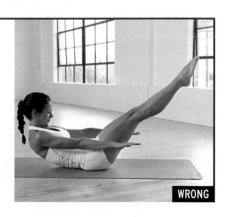

WRONG

Here's one ab shaper that will also teach you how to position your torso correctly.

THE RIGHT WAY

➤ Lie on your back with your feet off the floor and your knees bent; your legs should be slightly extended and your knees over your hips. Hold a resistance band stretched across the front of your thighs, without locking elbows.

➤ Slowly curl your torso until your shoulder blades are off the floor, concentrating on bringing your lower ribs in and down toward your navel.

➤ Using your abs, not your hip flexors, pull your hips toward your chest, slightly lifting your tailbone and buttocks off the floor. As your thighs move toward your chest, resist the band.

➤ Keep your eyes looking straight ahead and your spine rounded. Hold for four counts. Slowly lower your pelvis to the starting position.

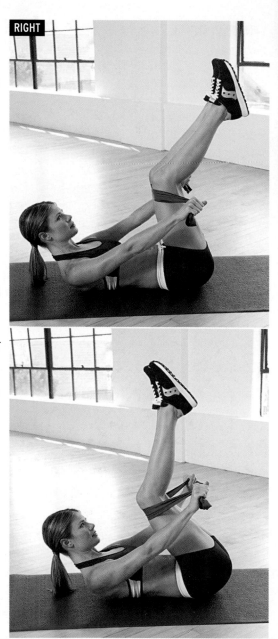

RIGHT

MUSCLES WORKED
rectus abdominis, transverse abdominis, external obliques, internal obliques

PELVIC LIFT AND CURL

THE PAYOFF
The pelvic lift and curl will teach you the basics of good posture, showing you how to use your abs to stabilize your torso and keep your spine in the proper position. Once you begin to practice good abdominal mechanics in your everyday movements, you'll really see the payoff from other ab work.

WORKOUT GUIDELINES
Do 1 to 2 sets of 8 reps, working your way up to 12 reps. Rest 45 to 60 seconds between sets. To progress, do the same moves, with legs straight, or increase the resistance by choking up on the band so it's tighter against your thighs.

EXPERT ADVICE
"If you don't have a resistance band, use a towel and press manually against your thighs," says Karen Clippinger, M.S.P.E., Los Angeles-based kinesiologist and instructor at UCLA. "Whether you're using a band or a towel as resistance, emphasize the ab work by contracting your abdominals as if you're trying to press your belly button against the floor."

The pelvic lift and curl will show you how to use your abs to stabilize your torso.

MISTAKES TO AVOID
➤ **Don't** use momentum or swing your legs over your head; this uses your back and hip flexor muscles to perform the curl, not your abs.
➤ **Don't** drop your head backward, placing stress on your cervical spine.
➤ **Don't** arch your back in the starting position. This puts stress on your lower-back muscles.

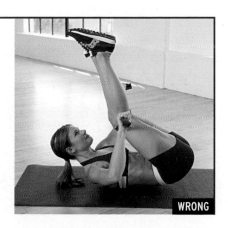

WRONG

Take the abdominal curl to new heights for stronger abs.

THE RIGHT WAY

➤ Tie a resistance band in a loop and put legs through it, resting it above knees. Lie on your back, knees bent at a 90-degree angle, and in line with hips. Drop tailbone so lower back touches floor. Place fingertips lightly on the sides of your head.

➤ Slowly lift head and curl torso upward. Then, reach your hands forward as far as possible, palms up, curling torso slightly higher, making sure shoulder blades clear the floor but the back portion of your waist is still in contact with the floor.

➤ Maintaining this position, tuck your pelvis and bring left knee toward chest, resisting the motion with the resistance band as you straighten right leg. Bend both knees, keeping torso even. Repeat for all reps.

MUSCLES WORKED
rectus abdominis, external obliques, internal obliques, transverse abdominis

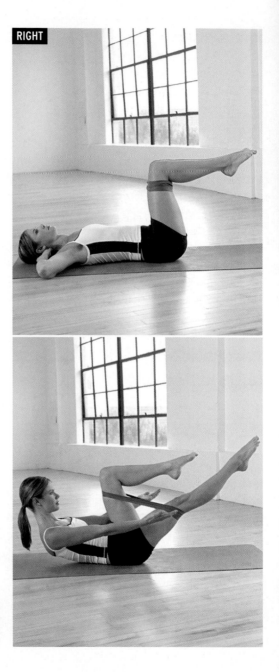

RIGHT

KNEE-TO-CHEST CURL

THE PAYOFF
This knee-to-chest curl delivers maximum results by working your abs using a band for resistance. During much of your day, your abs function as stabilizers to keep your back from arching excessively and your pelvis from tilting forward as you stand, sit or walk. This exercise emphasizes that stabilization role and trains the abs to perform properly.

WORKOUT GUIDELINES
Do 1 set of 8 reps on the right side, then 8 reps on the left. Rest 45 to 60 seconds after completing a set with each leg. Repeat for one more set on each side. Progress by increasing from 8 to 12 to 15 reps per side or lowering the extended leg more parallel to the floor, keeping back in full contact with the floor.

EXPERT ADVICE
"Focus on curling your ribs and pelvis toward your navel, pulling the abdominal wall inward," says Karen Clippinger, M.S.P.E., Los Angeles-based kinesiologist and instructor at UCLA. "Keep your torso as rounded as possible in the lifted position."

While basic curls work, this knee-to-chest curl delivers maximum results.

MISTAKES TO AVOID

➤ **Don't** lift your torso up too high or use momentum and allow your waist to leave the floor; this causes strain in your neck, shoulders, back and hip flexors.
➤ **Don't** let your back arch or your torso drop, stressing your back muscles.
➤ **Don't** perform quick "bicycling" movements with your legs; this may cause you to roll from side to side due to a loss of torso stability.

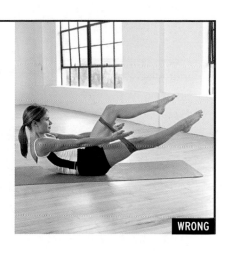

WRONG

One great yoga pose to tighten and tone your entire torso.

abdominals

THE RIGHT WAY

➤ Sit erect on your sit bones (at the base of your butt), knees bent, feet flat, and knees, ankles and feet together.
➤ Place hands behind thighs, contract abs and stay as erect as possible as you lift one leg at a time until calves are parallel to the floor, knees bent at a 90-degree angle.
➤ Keeping shoulders down and away from ears, chest lifted, shoulder blades down, continue to hold your thighs and straighten both legs out at about a 45-degree angle.
➤ Keep breathing evenly through your nose, holding pose for recommended breaths.
➤ Come out of the position by lowering feet to floor, keeping abs contracted throughout.

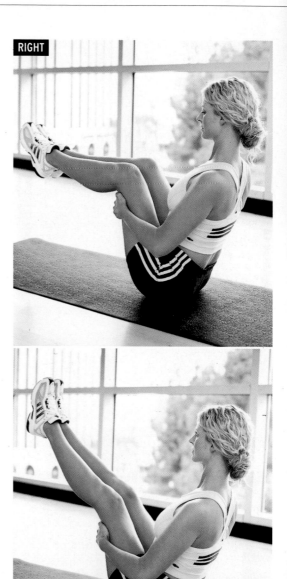

RIGHT

MUSCLES WORKED
rectus abdominis, external obliques, internal obliques, transverse abdominis, erector spinae

V-SIT

THE PAYOFF
This exercise effectively trains the opposing abdominal muscles and spine extensors to work together to keep you upright, creating better posture and core strength, flatter abs and a more beautiful back. It can also help you build the muscle endurance you need to perform more challenging exercises – not to mention almost any activity – more effectively.

WORKOUT GUIDELINES
Hold the pose for 5 breaths, then release and repeat one more time. To progress, hold for 6-8 breaths and repeat.

EXPERT ADVICE
"As you hold the V-sit position, think about lengthening your body up through the top of your head as well as opening and lifting your chest," says New York City-based Reebok University Master Trainer Lisa Wheeler. "This allows you to balance, stay erect and stabilize your torso so you work your abdominals most effectively."

This exercise trains the opposing abdominal muscles and spine extensors to work together to keep you upright.

MISTAKES TO AVOID

➤ **Don't** round your shoulders, curving the upper back; this causes destabilization of the spine, which can stress the upper back and shoulder muscles as well as delicate connective tissue in the spine.
➤ **Don't** lean back too far and slouch; this not only stresses your lower back, but also makes the exercise ineffective because you can't contract your abs.
➤ **Don't** pop out the ribs; this can force you into a hyperextended spine, preventing stabilization as well as exercise effectiveness.

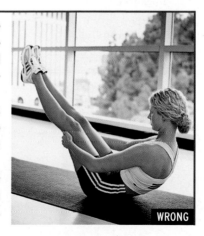

WRONG

Turn upside down for tighter abs and better posture.

THE RIGHT WAY

➤ Drape your body facedown over a stability ball, then walk hands forward until your knees and lower legs are resting on the ball, hands on the floor, elbows straight but not locked, shoulders in line with wrists.

➤ Tighten abdominal muscles to prevent low back from arching. Your shoulders, torso, pelvis, knees and ankles should form a straight line.

➤ Contract abs as you lift hips. Keeping head down, draw legs up so that your body forms an inverted V, with feet pressing against the ball.

➤ Pause for 4 counts; then slowly return to starting position. Use your abs to control the motion and keep low back from arching.

MUSCLES WORKED
rectus abdominis, external obliques, transverse abdominis, internal obliques, iliopsoas

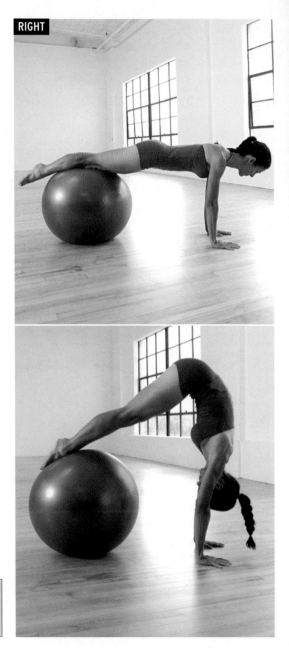

RIGHT

INVERTED V

THE PAYOFF
The inverted V works your entire abdominal area, engaging the lower portion of your abs more completely than the traditional crunch. The results are tighter abs and better posture, which can prevent back pain. You'll learn to keep your spine in its natural position while your arms and legs are moving.

WORKOUT GUIDELINES
Do 1 set of 6 reps; work up to 12. When you can do 12 with good form, either add a second set, or start with only your ankles and feet supported by the ball and lift your pelvis higher (you'll work through a larger range of motion). Drop back to 6 reps and gradually work back up to 12.

EXPERT ADVICE
"Initiate the movement by using your abdominals rather than just pulling the ball with your legs," says Karen Clippinger, M.S.P.E., a Los Angeles-based kinesiologist and instructor at UCLA. "Once in the inverted position, use the same abdominal control to roll the ball away from you."

The inverted V works your abdominal area more completely than the traditional crunch.

MISTAKES TO AVOID

➤ **Don't** pike and overshoot your shoulders; this strains your shoulder, wrist and neck muscles.
➤ **Don't** let your belly sag in the starting position; it will be difficult to lift your hips in the V and will also stress back muscles.
➤ **Don't** lift your head up; this puts pressure on the delicate connective tissue in your neck.

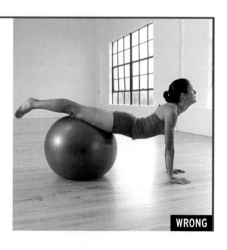

WRONG

Tighten, tone and whittle your middle — no mat work required.

THE RIGHT WAY

➤ Attach 2 ab straps to secure hanging hooks, slightly more than shoulder-width apart, and place a box or bench on the floor to help you get into position.

➤ Slip upper arms through straps so they're just above elbows; hold straps.

➤ Bend and lift knees so thighs are parallel to floor; ankles are in line with knees.

➤ With shoulder blades squeezed together and down, contract abs, exhale and slowly curl pelvis up and in, drawing navel to spine.

➤ Continue curl until abs feel fully contracted; thighs will lift slightly, and will tuck under. Release slowly to start position; repeat.

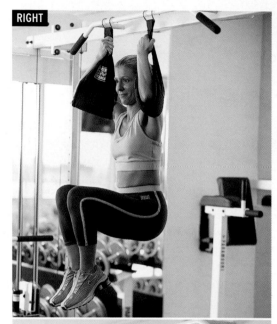

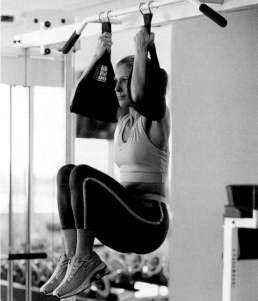

MUSCLES WORKED
rectus abdominis, external obliques, internal obliques, transverse abdominis

HANGING REVERSE CRUNCH

THE PAYOFF
This isolation move targets the muscle fibers of your lower abdominal region, yielding a firmer, more toned midsection. By strengthening the lower portion of your abs, you'll learn how to control the tendency to arch your back, which is crucial to maintaining posture and alignment. It promotes more mobility in your pelvis, priming you for sports, exercise and many everyday activities.

WORKOUT GUIDELINES
Begin with 1 set of 10-15 reps, pro- gressing to 25 reps. When you can do 25 with good form, add a second set, beginning with 15, pro- gressing up to 25. Rest 60 seconds between sets.

EXPERT ADVICE
"Once you're in the starting posi- tion, focus the action entirely on the area between the ribs and the top of the pelvis," says Douglas Brooks, M.S., a consulting exercise physiologist and personal trainer based in Northern California. "This region is where all of the movement occurs; no other part of your body should be stirring."

This move targets the muscle fibers of your lower abdominal region, yielding a firmer midsection.

MISTAKES TO AVOID

➤ **Don't** swing torso or kick legs up; this puts stress on the hip flexors and causes your back to hyperextend.
➤ **Don't** drop knees below 90 degrees; this puts stress on the lower back, and your abs will do less work.
➤ **Don't** let your upper back round; this will strain the neck and shoulders and minimize the abdominal efficiency.

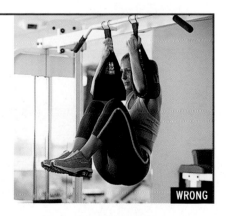

WRONG

ARM EXERCISES

arms

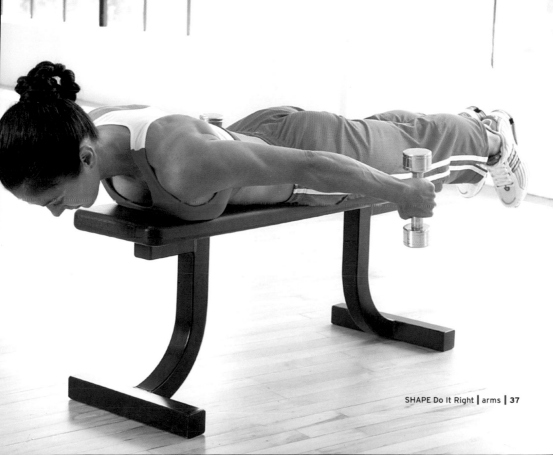

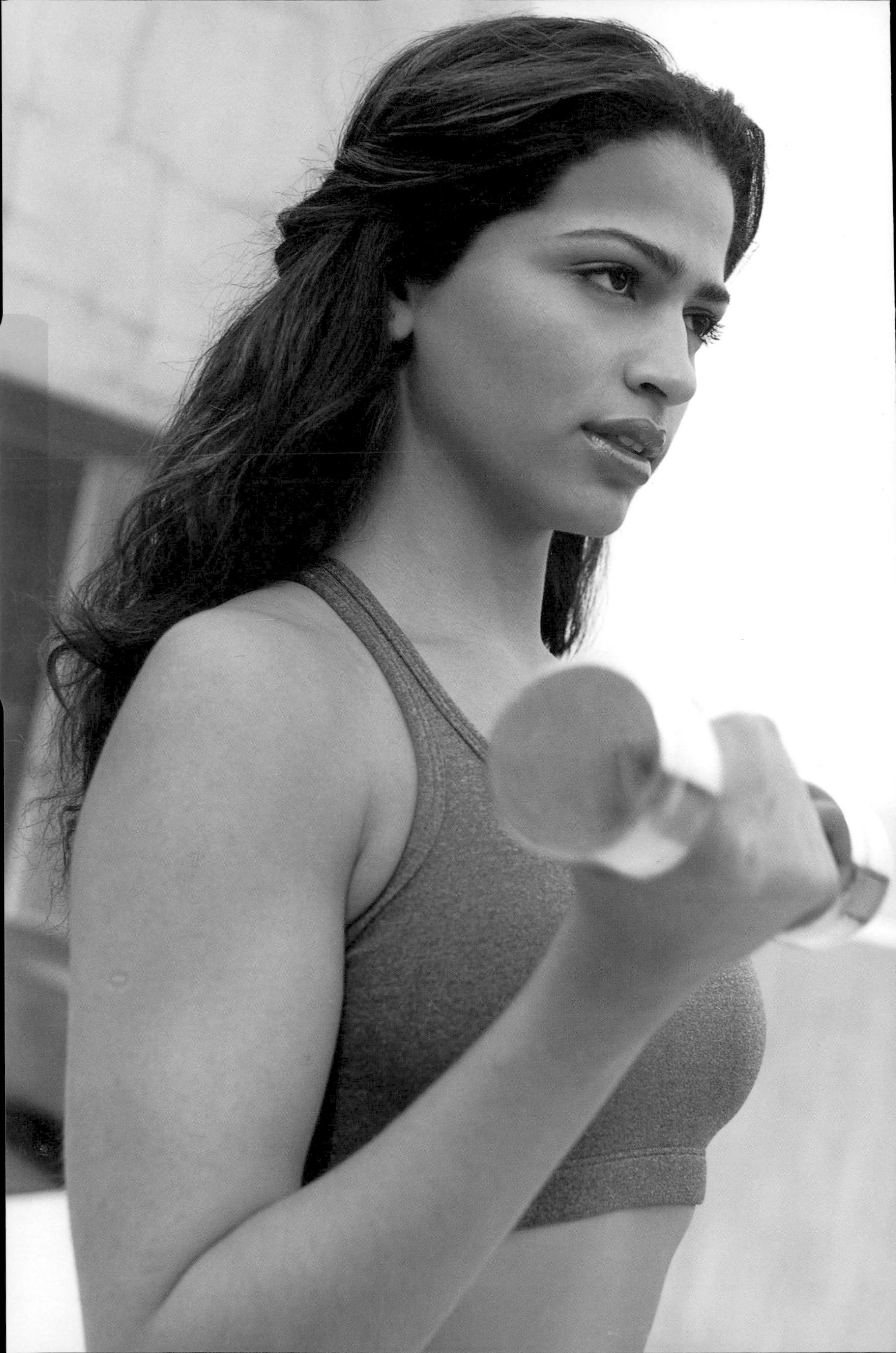

ARMS

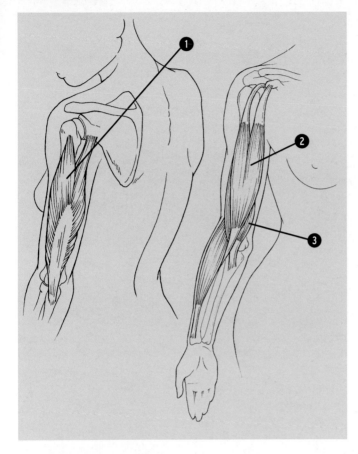

MUSCLES
1. triceps brachii
2. biceps brachii
3. brachialis

The biceps brachii and brachialis – the muscles on the front of your upper arm – flex the elbow and rotate the forearm so your palms can face upward or downward. The biceps has a long head and a short head. Both cross the shoulder joint at different places, attach on the shoulder blade and insert together just below your elbow joint on the forearm. The brachialis lies under the biceps and crosses only your elbow joint.

The triceps muscle is on the rear of your upper arm. It is one muscle comprised of three sections, joined together in one common tendon below the elbow. Together the lateral, medial and long heads extend your elbow to straighten your arm. Both the lateral and medial heads originate on the upper arm bone (humerus) and the long head crosses the shoulder joint, attaching on the shoulder blade.

Create upper-body strength for your favorite activities.

THE RIGHT WAY

➤ Hold a dumbbell in each hand with arms by your sides, elbows in line with shoulders and palms forward. Stand with your feet about hip-width apart, legs straight, but not locked.

➤ Contract your abdominals, bringing spine to a neutral position. With chest lifted and shoulders squared, look straight ahead, not down.

➤ Keeping your elbows at your sides and your upper arms still, bend both elbows and slowly lift the dumbbells. Focus on bringing your wrists in toward your shoulders. At the top of the motion, with the meaty part of your forearm touching your biceps, your knuckles should face the ceiling.

➤ Slowly straighten arms to starting position without changing elbow or shoulder position.

MUSCLES WORKED
biceps, brachialis

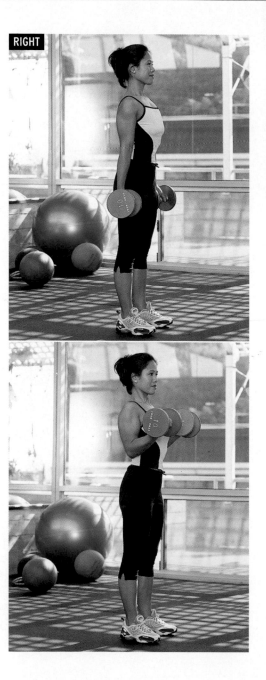

BICEPS CURL

THE PAYOFF
This is the move to get you strong, firm biceps, which translate into extra power for pulling motions such as rock climbing and rowing – and a great look in cap sleeves and tank tops. Your biceps muscle is one of the first muscles to show shape and definition from very little training; a light weight goes a long way. As an added bonus, you'll increase your forearm strength for a more powerful grip on a tennis racket, giving more power to your swing.

WORKOUT GUIDELINES
Do 1 or 2 sets of 12-15 reps, eventually adding a third set. Rest 60 seconds between sets. To progress, advanced lifters may want to add this exercise in as part of an upper-body superset. Use 5- to 10-pound dumbbells in each hand.

EXPERT ADVICE
"Focus on driving your upper forearm into your biceps, as if there's a walnut in the crease of your elbow," says Chicago-based trainer Mark Cibrario. "As you curl, imagine trying to crack the nut open."

This is the move to get you strong, firm biceps, which translate into extra power for pulling motions.

MISTAKES TO AVOID
➤ **Don't** arch your back or scoot your pelvis forward. Mistakes like these can overstress the ligaments and muscles in your lower back.

➤ **Don't** let your upper arm move forward or behind your torso; you'll engage your front shoulder muscles and cheat your biceps out of a good workout.

➤ **Don't** "cock" your wrist backward or try and get more biceps work by curling your wrist upward.

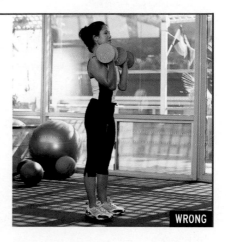

WRONG

If you want to effectively target your upper arms, take a seat.

THE RIGHT WAY

➤ Hold a dumbbell in your left hand and sit on a chair, feet flat on floor and separated slightly wider than hip-width apart, ankles aligned with knees.

➤ Lean forward from your hips, keeping back straight and in a neutral position. Place rear of left upper arm firmly against left inner thigh so your left arm hangs toward the floor in line with left shoulder, wrist in a neutral position with palm facing in; place right hand on right thigh for support.

➤ Contract abdominals to maintain a neutral spine, keep chest open and shoulders relaxed.

➤ Maintain position and bend left elbow, bringing dumbbell up toward left shoulder; pause, squeezing biceps at the top of the movement.

➤ Slowly lower to starting position until elbow is straight but not locked.

MUSCLES WORKED
biceps, brachialis

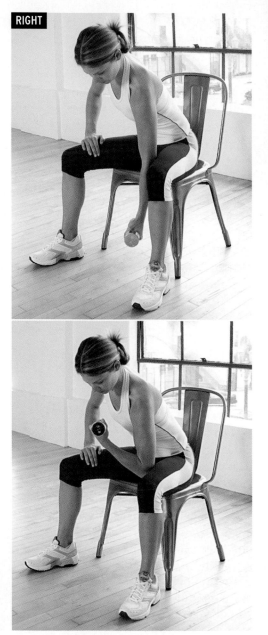

RIGHT

CONCENTRATION CURL

THE PAYOFF
The supported position of the concentration curl effectively isolates your biceps. You'll glean defined and toned upper arms while lessening the chance to swing your arms or hyperextend your elbows, two exercise errors that severely decrease efficiency. Buff biceps are important assets when it comes to tasks such as lifting and carrying.

WORKOUT GUIDELINES
Do 1 to 2 sets of 8 to 12 alternating reps. (One set equals both arms.)

Use as much weight as you can to fatigue by 12 reps. To progress, increase weight in 1- to 3-pound increments. Use 5 to 20 pounds.

EXPERT ADVICE:
"Focus on keeping your wrist in a neutral position and your middle finger in line with the middle of your wrist," says Karen Clippinger, M.S.P.E., a Los Angeles-based kinesiologist and teacher at UCLA. "This aligns the dumbbell at the correct angle to your shoulder, honing in on your biceps more effectively."

Buff biceps are important assets when it comes to tasks such as lifting and carrying.

MISTAKES TO AVOID

➤ **Don't** place elbow on top of thigh instead of resting on inside of thigh. This may cause your arm to slip which is inefficient and dangerous, especially if you're using a heavy weight.
➤ **Don't** let your wrist "cock" backward, which places a lot of strain on the forearm and wrist connective tissue.
➤ **Don't** hunch your shoulders or round your back; this lessens torso stability for lifting the weight even though your arm is braced.

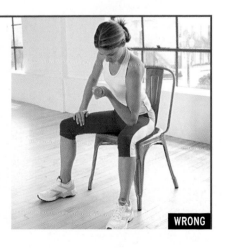

WRONG

Lose the arm flab and get a strong, firm torso to boot.

THE RIGHT WAY

➤ Stand or kneel (depending on machine) on foot plate with knees (or feet) directly under hips.

➤ Place hands on the lower bars and straighten your arms. If the machine has the option, turn bars in closer toward your body.

➤ Contract your abdominal muscles and squeeze your shoulder blades down and together. Don't lock your elbows.

➤ Lower the foot plate by bending your elbows, keeping them pointing straight back until hands align with your upper hips or lower ribs, shoulders are still pulled back.

➤ Press your body back up, straightening arms, and repeat the movement.

MUSCLES WORKED
triceps

RIGHT

ASSISTED TRI-DIP

THE PAYOFF
The gravity-assisted machine lets you use the optimum amount of resistance to challenge your entire upper torso with enough weight, which is difficult to do when using body weight only. The machine also helps you to maintain a smooth lifting and lowering pattern and improves your form for firmer triceps and shapelier shoulders. Your chest, back and abdominal muscles will be stronger, too.

WORKOUT GUIDELINES
Set the machine to your body weight minus 20-40 pounds (the more weight you use, the easier it is) and do 1 to 2 sets of 12-15 reps to fatigue, resting 45 to 60 seconds between sets. To progress, decrease the weight or add another set.

EXPERT ADVICE
"Keep your body perfectly straight from head to knees (or heels) throughout the exercise," says Evanston, Ill., strength and conditioning specialist CC Cunningham, M.S. "This forces your triceps to do most of the work instead of relying on the power of your torso."

The gravity-assisted machine lets you use the optimum amount of resistance and improves your form.

MISTAKES TO AVOID

➤ **Don't** roll your shoulders forward; this can stress shoulder joints and upper-back muscles.
➤ **Don't** point your elbows out; this can reduce the amount of work your triceps are doing.
➤ **Don't** let your body drop so low that your hands reach higher than your lower ribs; this will prevent you from being able to straighten your arms to press back up.

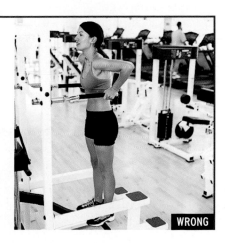

WRONG

Discover the power of the press in your quest for toned upper arms.

THE RIGHT WAY

➤ Lying on a flat bench, knees bent and feet on bench edge, hold a dumbbell in each hand. Keep elbows bent and pointing up, dumbbells level with your ears, thumbs pointing down.

➤ Contract abdominals, bringing spine to a neutral position and in contact with bench. Squeeze shoulder blades down and away from ears.

➤ Keeping upper arms still, straighten arms and press the dumbbells upward in a controlled manner as you gradually rotate your forearms so that your palms face forward when your arms are fully straightened. Pause briefly at the top of the movement.

➤ Point your thumbs behind you, rotate your forearms back and slowly lower the weights to the starting position. Repeat.

MUSCLES WORKED
triceps

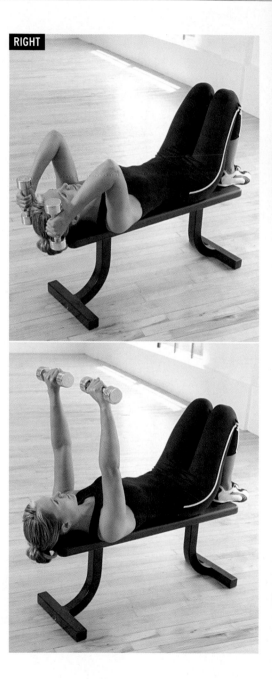

RIGHT

LYING OVERHEAD EXTENSION

THE PAYOFF

Weak triceps and lack of muscle tone add little shape to the rear of your upper arm. To develop toned and taut triceps, try this overhead triceps extension, which emphasizes the inner portion of the triceps muscle. You'll give svelte shape to your upper arms and shoulders and at the same time develop strength, helpful for any pushing movement.

WORKOUT GUIDELINES

Do 2 to 3 sets of 10 to 15 reps as part of your regular training program, resting 45 to 60 seconds between sets. To progress, increase your weight in 2-pound increments. Use 5 to 10 pounds in each hand to start.

EXPERT ADVICE

"Think about squeezing elbows together and at the same time, drawing shoulder blades down your back," says Los Angeles-based certified trainer Keli Roberts, ACE spokesperson and Group Fitness Manager at Equinox in Pasadena, Calif. "This keeps the upper arm from moving while straightening and bending the elbows."

To develop toned triceps, try this overhead extension, which emphasizes the inner portion of the triceps muscle.

MISTAKES TO AVOID

➤ **Don't** let your elbows point outward or inward as this can place stress on elbow tendons as you straighten your arms.
➤ **Don't** drop your arms so far behind it causes you to arch your back, taking you out of a neutral and protected spine position.
➤ **Don't** move your wrists even though your forearm is rotating; this may strain the forearm and the wrist's connective tissue.

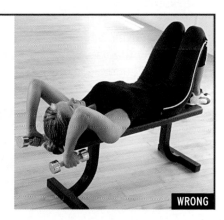

WRONG

You'll get noticeable results from this classic triceps toner.

THE RIGHT WAY

➤ With your back to a chair, place hands on edge of the seat so wrists align with shoulders. Fingers point forward, arms are straight but not locked, knees bent and feet flat on floor slightly ahead of your knees.

➤ Squeeze your shoulder blades down and together, chest lifted and shoulders relaxed so you can support yourself with your arms.

➤ Contract abdominals so spine is in a neutral position with back, and buttocks is close to chair seat.

➤ Slowly bend elbows without flaring them outward by lowering hips toward the floor, going only as far as you can without lifting shoulders or rolling them forward; don't exceed a 90-degree angle at your elbows.

➤ Press back up to starting position, slowly straightening arms without locking them.

MUSCLES WORKED
triceps, anterior deltoid, pectoralis major

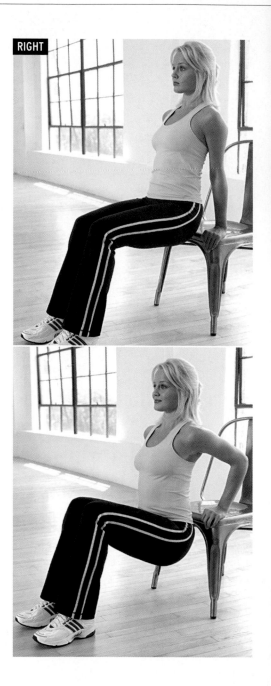

RIGHT

CHAIR DIP

THE PAYOFF
The chair dip is a great way to challenge your upper arms, plus a well-executed dip also works the upper-back muscles to improve posture and prevent shoulder problems. As an added benefit to firm triceps, the chest muscles, which are commonly tight, will get a dynamic stretch, as well as a different range of strengthening.

WORKOUT GUIDELINES
Do 1 set of 8 reps, working up to 12. When you can do 12 reps with correct form, add another set of 8 reps and work up to 12. Rest 60 seconds between sets. To progress, when you can do 2 sets of 12 reps comfortably, perform the exercise with legs farther out in front of you, balanced on your heels.

EXPERT ADVICE
"Concentrate on pressing your palms down as if you're pushing through the chair seat through the entire exercise," says Karen Clippinger, M.S.P.E., a Los Angeles-based kinesiologist and teacher at UCLA. "This ensures you'll use your arms to do the work, not your legs."

A well-executed dip also works upper-back muscles to improve posture and prevent shoulder problems.

MISTAKES TO AVOID
➤ **Don't** let your back and butt drift away from the chair seat; this takes the work away from your arms and can also place strain on your back.
➤ **Don't** dip down too low; You run the risk of straining your neck and shoulder muscles.
➤ **Don't** lock your elbows; this places tension on the elbow joints and can eventually lead to repetitive stress syndrome.

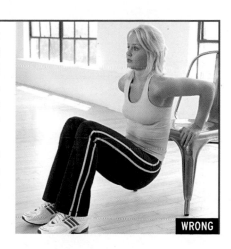

WRONG

Say goodbye to arms that keep waving when your hand stops. This move will banish the jiggle.

THE RIGHT WAY

➤ Holding a dumbbell in each hand, lie facedown on a flat bench with shoulders at bench edge, head extended over the edge, legs straight.

➤ Bend elbows so arms form 90-degree angles, upper arms parallel to back, wrists aligned with elbows, palms in and knuckles pointing toward floor; contract abs to bring spine to a neutral position.

➤ Squeeze shoulder blades down and together and slightly lift chest, being careful not to arch your back or lower elbows below waist level.

➤ From this position, extend both arms until elbows are straight but not locked, pausing briefly at the top of the movement. Slowly bend elbows to return to start position.

MUSCLES WORKED
triceps

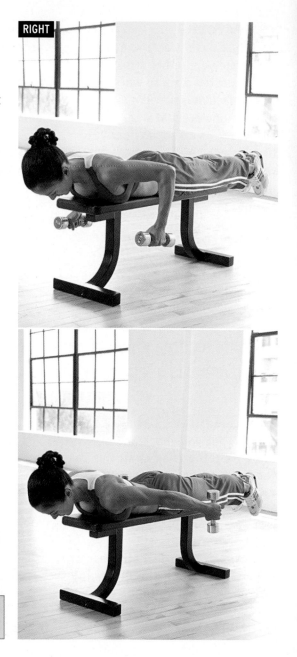

RIGHT

PRONE TRICEPS EXTENSION

THE PAYOFF

Think about the last time you waved at someone. When your hand stopped moving, did your upper arm continue? For ever-firm and jiggle-free upper arms, try this lying down version of the classic kickback. The prone position better allows you to maintain spine alignment and keep the rest of your body still so you can focus solely on toning your triceps.

WORKOUT GUIDELINES

Do 1 to 2 sets of 8-12 reps, resting 45-60 seconds between sets. When 12 reps are no longer challenging, gradually increase the resistance in 2-pound increments, to as much as 10 pounds per hand. To further progress, add a third set.

EXPERT ADVICE

"Focus on extending the elbows and wrists so the hands are at the same level as the elbows in the finished position," says Mission Viejo, Calif.-based certified trainer Rob Glick, B.S., Exercise Science and Regional Group Fitness Director for Crunch Fitness. "This ensures you're fully engaging the triceps through the last degrees of extension."

The prone position better allows you to maintain spine alignment and keep the rest of your body still.

MISTAKES TO AVOID

➤ **Don't** lift your arms so far behind you that it strains your shoulders and back; the weight of the dumbbells is pulling downward on your muscles.

➤ **Don't** perform the move so quickly that you snap your elbows; this may result in tendon and ligament strain in your elbows.

➤ **Don't** lift your head. This can place excess strain on your cervical spine, especially when you're pressing the weights behind you.

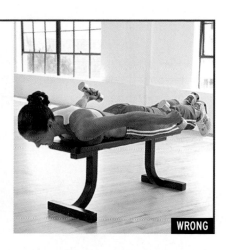

WRONG

Get shapely arms in one simple, clean sweep.

THE RIGHT WAY

➤ Holding a dumbbell in your right hand, kneel with your left knee resting on a bench, left arm straight and left palm flat on bench.

➤ Bend right knee slightly and make sure your back is parallel to the floor, maintaining a natural arch in your lower back. Keep your shoulders square and your head in line with your spine. Contract your abs by pulling your navel toward your spine.

➤ Bend right arm up and behind you so that upper arm is near torso and parallel to the floor, palm facing in.

➤ Keeping upper arm stationary and squeezed against your ribs, extend elbow until arm is straight. Slowly return to the starting position.

MUSCLES WORKED
triceps

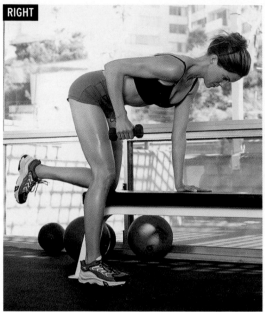

RIGHT

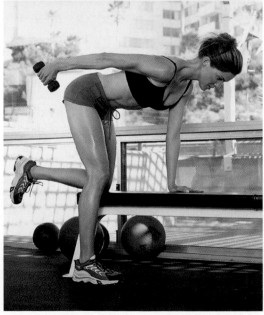

TRICEPS KICKBACK

THE PAYOFF
You'll say goodbye to undeveloped upper arms, create a beautiful curve and enjoy new strength with this classic triceps exercise. By using a bench for support, you have to rely on abdominal and back core strength to maintain the bentover position, which allows you to get full extension of your upper arm for toned and tightened triceps without strain.

WORKOUT GUIDELINES
Do 3 sets of alternating 12 reps (1 set equals reps with both arms) with a 5- to 10-pound dumbbell.

To progress, increase your weight in 2-pound increments or super-set this move with another triceps exercise.

EXPERT ADVICE
"If possible, perform this move sideways next to a mirror so you can watch your posture and alignment," says Los Angeles-based certified trainer Keli Roberts, ACE spokesperson and Group Fitness Manager at Equinox in Pasadena, Calif. "Most people don't have good body awareness, and it's easy to make mistakes."

You'll say goodbye to undeveloped upper arms and enjoy new strength with this classic triceps exercise.

MISTAKES TO AVOID
➤ **Don't** swing your upper arm. This engages your shoulder muscles and shifts work away from your triceps.
➤ **Don't** raise your right shoulder and upper back and dip to your left. These errors place excess stress on your neck and back muscles, while decreasing the exercise's effectiveness.
➤ **Don't** use so much weight that you're unable to straighten your arm fully.

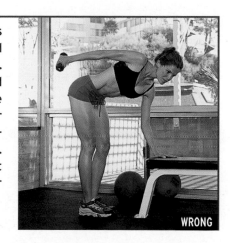

WRONG

BACK EXERCISES

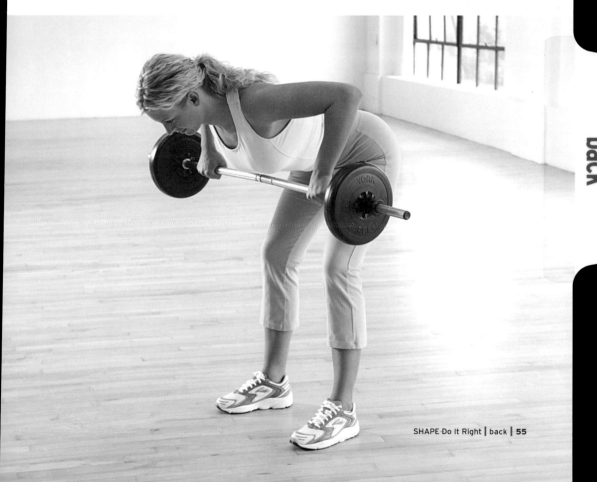

back

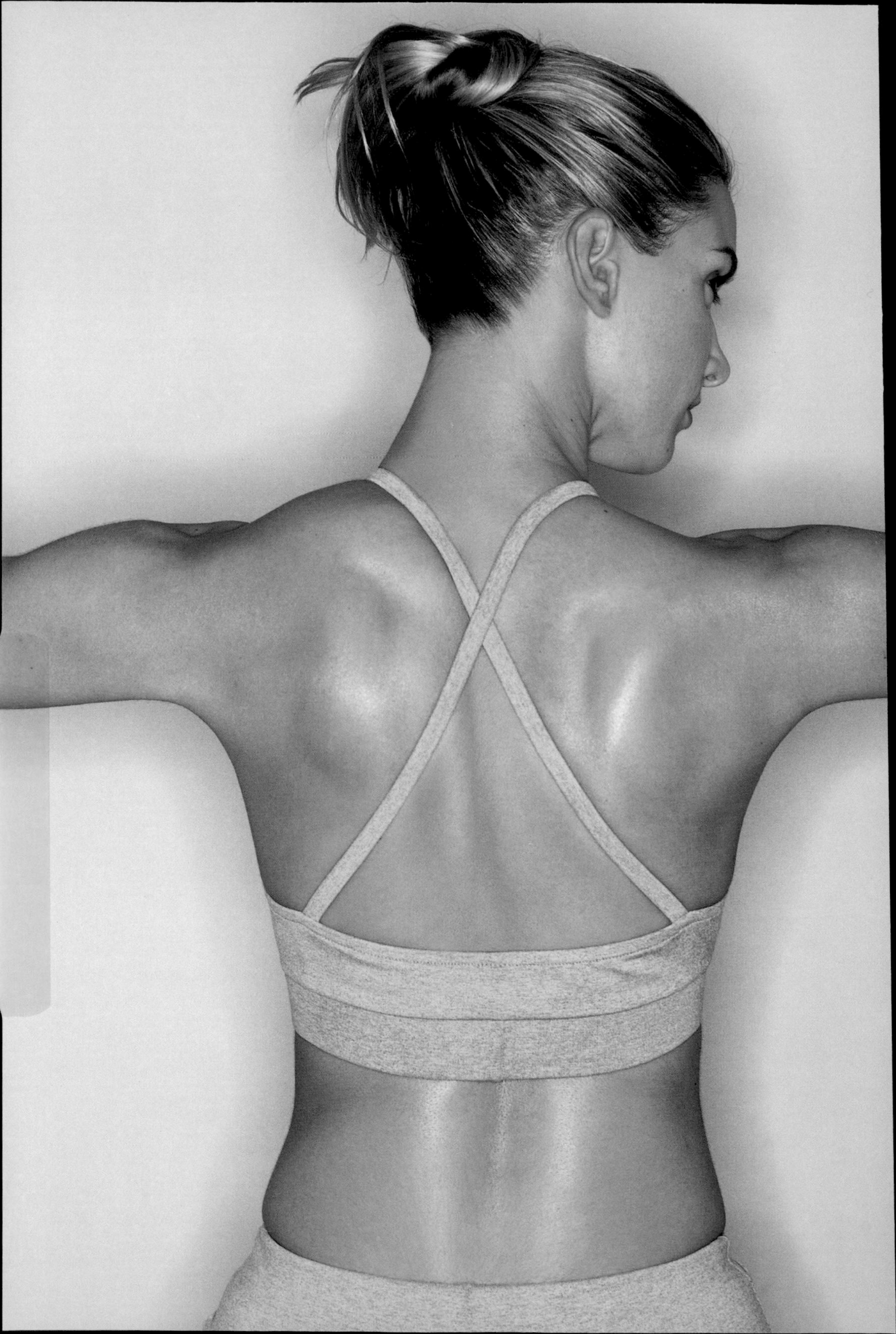

BACK

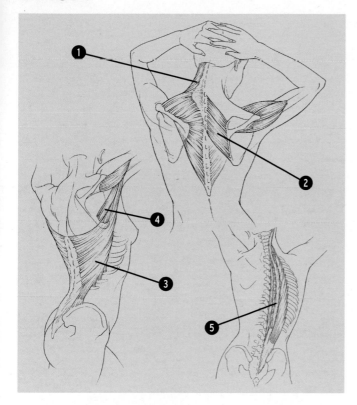

MUSCLES
1. trapezius
2. rhomboids
3. latissimus dorsi
4. teres major
5. erector spinae

The trapezius and rhomboid muscles make up your upper back. The trapezius attaches to the base of your skull, midback vertebrae and either end of your collarbone. The upper portion is involved in overhead pushing actions; the middle draws your shoulder blades back; and the lower region draws your arms back. The rhomboids lie horizontally underneath the trapezius, pulling your shoulder blades back and down.

The latissimus dorsi (plural: lats) covers the lower and middle portions of the back. It originates on the spine, at the top of the hipbone, and attaches to the upper arm. The lats move the upper arm downward, pull the elbows down and inward, and the arms behind you, and assist the shoulders with inward rotation. Teres major, a small muscle attaching on the inside of the shoulder blade, performs the same movements.

The spine extensors are three muscle pairs, collectively known as the erector spinae. They run from hip to neck on either side of your spine, branching off to attach at the ribs and spine.

Make your waist look smaller – and stand straighter – with one move.

THE RIGHT WAY

➤ Set weight (see "Workout Guidelines") and stand (or kneel) on an assisted pull-up machine. Feet (or knees) should be in line with shoulders. Hold parallel grips, palms facing in and above slightly bent elbows.

➤ Contract abdominal muscles so spine is naturally curved, and pull shoulder blades down and away from ears. Maintain downward squeeze and tightened abs for the entire exercise to keep torso from swinging.

➤ Maintaining shoulder-blade position, elbows in front, start to pull yourself up.

➤ Drive elbows toward your waist as you lift; finish with elbows pointing down. Slowly straighten arms, without changing torso alignment; repeat.

MUSCLES WORKED
latissimus dorsi, teres major, posterior deltoid

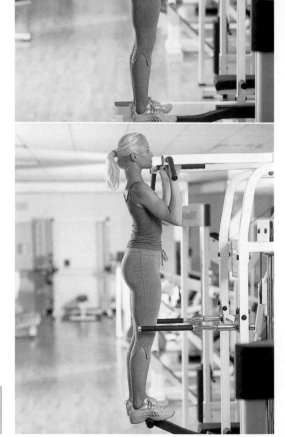

RIGHT

ASSISTED PULL-UP

THE PAYOFF
More than creating a beautiful V-shape to your back and improving your posture, the machine is the biggest advantage with this move. You'll be able to do pull-ups correctly, regardless of your fitness level, because the machine assists you in lifting a percentage of your body weight. By varying grips, you can fully work your largest back muscles and shoulders, building them so your waist and hips look smaller.

WORKOUT GUIDELINES
Do 1-2 sets of 15-20 reps, resting 60 seconds between sets. Lift about 60-70 percent of your body weight. To progress, or if you're a seasoned lifter: Do 2-3 sets of 15-20 reps and change your grip for variety.

EXPERT ADVICE
"Use your back muscles, not your biceps to pull yourself," says Douglas Brooks, M.S., a Northern California exercise physiologist and personal trainer. "Before you begin, press your lat muscles downward (but don't bend your elbows), and concentrate on working them as you lift."

The machine assists you in lifting only a percentage of your body weight.

MISTAKES TO AVOID
➤ **Don't** pull your elbows behind you. This can place stress on the front of the shoulder muscles and doesn't increase the challenge of the exercise.
➤ **Don't** lock your elbows in the starting position; it adds unnecessary mechanical stress to the elbow joint.
➤ **Don't** swing your body as you pull up, or you can lose alignment and decrease the effectiveness of the move.

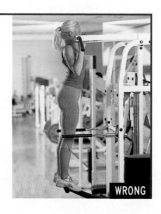

WRONG

Sculpt a strong, sexy silhouette and improve your posture.

THE RIGHT WAY

➤ Attach a V-shaped bar to a low-cable pulley. Sit erect on bench with feet on support plate separated hip-width apart, knees slightly bent, toes pointing up. Hinge forward from your hips to grasp bar at mid-abdomen level, hands slightly less than shoulder-width apart, arms straight, palms facing in. Sit erect again to begin.

➤ Contract abdominals, bringing spine to a neutral position. Draw shoulder blades down and together.

➤ Bend elbows back and toward waist, pulling bar to rib cage.

➤ Straighten arms and return to starting position, maintaining torso alignment. Chest is lifted and shoulders are down throughout the entire movement.

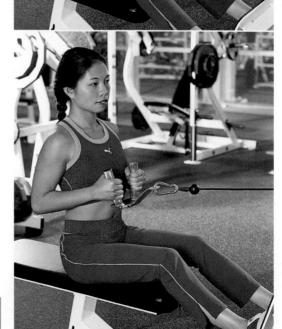

RIGHT

MUSCLES WORKED
latissimus dorsi, teres major, posterior deltoid

SEATED CABLE ROW

THE PAYOFF

This move strengthens and tones the powerful muscles of your middle back, making your waist and hips appear more slender. Strong lats will also put more oomph in your tennis or golf swing and help counteract that slumped posture common among runners and cyclists. As a bonus, you'll work your biceps and rear shoulder muscles.

WORKOUT GUIDELINES

Do 2 or 3 sets of 10-12 reps, lifting 30-60 pounds, depending on the machine. Rest 60 seconds between sets. To progress, increase your weight in 10-pound increments, or, change your bar for variety.

EXPERT ADVICE

"To protect your back, pay as much attention to getting yourself into position as you do to the mechanics of the exercise," says Juan Carlos Santana, M.Ed., C.S.C.S., owner of Optimum Performance Systems in Boca Raton, Fla. "With proper set-up, you'll be able to maintain the alignment necessary to target your back muscles without any spine stress."

Pay as much attention to getting yourself into position as you do to the mechanics of the exercise.

MISTAKES TO AVOID

➤ **Don't** straighten your legs or round your back when you reach forward to grasp the bar. The bent-leg position protects your lower back.
➤ **Don't** shrug your shoulders as you start to pull. You'll lose stabilization in the shoulder joint and put your rotator-cuff muscles at risk for injury.
➤ **Don't** lean back beyond the point at which your torso is perpendicular to the floor. Otherwise, the move will become more of a shoulder exercise.

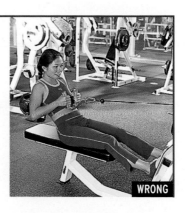

WRONG

Get a stronger spine, add balance to your muscles and prevent injury in just one move.

THE RIGHT WAY

➤ Stand on the platform of a 45-degree hyperextension bench, feet hip-width apart, legs straight and knees soft. Grasp handles and slide forward, facedown, until hips are completely supported on the pad with torso hanging off.

➤ Contract abdominals and bend forward, keeping spine neutral, and let head, neck and torso hang down. Cross arms over chest, hands on opposite shoulders.

➤ Maintaining abdominal tension, use lower back muscles to slowly raise torso until body is upright (normal posture). Keep head in line with spine and squeeze shoulder blades down and back, so chest is open. Hold briefly, then slowly lower torso, keeping hips against pad.

MUSCLES WORKED
erector spinae

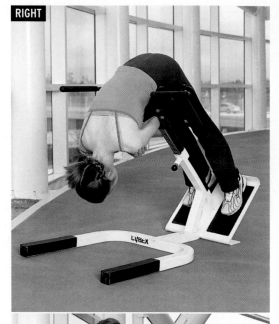

RIGHT

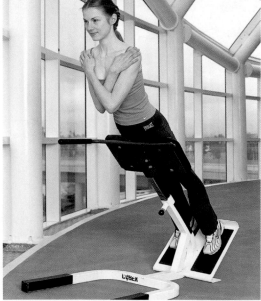

BACK EXTENSION ON BENCH

THE PAYOFF
This move strengthens the muscles and connective tissue that run along your spine and adds balance to your back muscles, so you'll avoid injury and have a solid foundation for almost any activity.

WORKOUT GUIDELINES
Do 1-3 sets of 8-15 reps, resting 30-60 seconds between sets. When you can complete 15 reps comfortably, try for more resistance by placing your hands behind your head or, for the biggest challenge, stretch your arms straight overhead.

EXPERT ADVICE
"Maintain equal tension between your abdominal and back muscles throughout the lift to help maintain your spine's natural curves," says Los Angeles-based certified trainer Keli Roberts, ACE spokesperson and Group Fitness Manager at Equinox in Pasadena, Calif. "In the finished position, you should look almost the same as when you're standing up."

This move strengthens the muscles and connective tissue that run along your spine.

MISTAKES TO AVOID

➤ **Don't** move too fast. Use your back muscles instead of momentum, or you'll lose the strengthening benefit and may even compress your spinal disks.
➤ **Don't** place added tension on your back by rounding it, then lifting up and arching backward or going beyond an upright, normal posture.
➤ **Don't** change arm positions until you're truly ready, or you may compromise your form and do the exercise incorrectly.

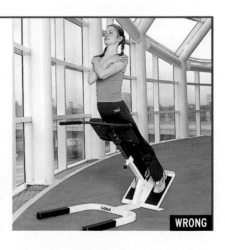

WRONG

Get a stronger, healthier and more beautiful upper body by perfecting this classic pose.

THE RIGHT WAY

➤ Lie facedown with legs extended and separated slightly, tops of feet and forearms on floor, hands flat and palms down, elbows bent and wrists in line with shoulders.

➤ Rest forehead on floor, relax shoulders, and pull belly up and in, dropping tailbone to a neutral position.

➤ Roll shoulders back and down, engaging back muscles to make space between shoulders and ears. Maintaining lifted belly, inhale and press palms against floor as you feel rib cage pull forward; lift head and chest without arching your back.

➤ Keep front of pelvis and pubic bone in contact with the floor, elbows bent and lifted, shoulders relaxed.

➤ Exhale, slowly lower to start position and repeat.

MUSCLES WORKED
erector spinae

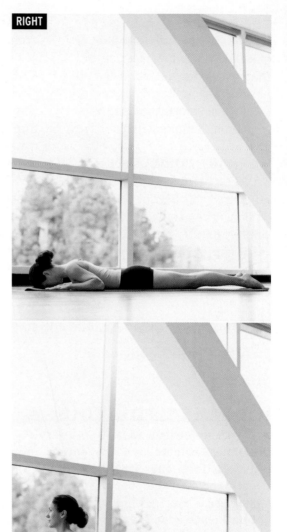

RIGHT

COBRA

THE PAYOFF
This classic yoga backbend strengthens the muscles that extend along your entire spine and increases spine mobility. It also opens up the chest and front of the shoulders, creating balance between the front and back of your torso, and it improves posture.

WORKOUT GUIDELINES
Do the move vinyasa, or flow, style: Inhale as you lift in 4 counts, then exhale and lower in 4 counts; repeat 3-4 times. To progress: On the last rep, hold lifted position for 3-5 breaths, then release. To increase the challenge, walk hands back, so forearms are off floor to start, elbows bent and lifted.

EXPERT ADVICE
"Think about lifting and opening your chest as if you were trying to pull your body forward and up off the floor," says New York City-based Reebok University Master Trainer Lisa Wheeler. "This will further activate the upper- and middle-back muscles and relieve pressure from the lower back while increasing strength."

This classic yoga backbend strengthens the muscles that extend along your entire spine.

MISTAKES TO AVOID
➤ **Don't** hyperextend into the lower back; this compresses the vertebrae and discs of the lower spine.
➤ **Don't** jam your shoulders up to your ears; this creates tension in your neck and shoulders, as well as an imbalance between the front and rear muscles of your torso.
➤ **Don't** release your abdominal control; this creates additional lower-back tension and discomfort.

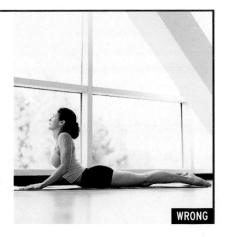

WRONG

Create a sexy, slimmer silhouette with the front lat pull-down.

back

THE RIGHT WAY

➤ Attach a long bar to a high-pulley cable.

➤ Sit to adjust the pad so that it rests on top of your thighs while your feet are flat on the floor.

➤ Stand and grasp the bar with an overhand grip and your hands slightly wider than shoulder-width apart. Take a seat, leaning back so the bar lines up with breastbone. Lean from your hips, not your lower back.

➤ Pull your shoulder blades down and back. Keeping your chest lifted, inhale, then exhale as you contract lats to pull the bar down, bending elbows down toward waist until bar is about 2 inches above your chest and your elbows point down. Slowly return bar to the starting position.

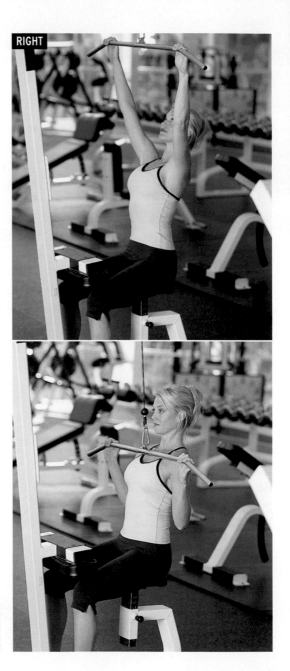

RIGHT

MUSCLES WORKED
latissimus dorsi , teres major, posterior deltoid

FRONT LAT PULL-DOWN

THE PAYOFF
This exercise tones and strengthens your latissimus dorsi, the large muscle that runs from behind each armpit to the center of your lower back. Training this muscle not only improves your posture but also widens your back, making your waist appear smaller.

WORKOUT GUIDELINES
Perform 2-3 sets of 8-12 reps, lifting 40-70 pounds. Rest 45 seconds between sets. To progress, increase weight or change to a close grip or angled bar for variety.

EXPERT ADVICE
"Remember that the lat pull-down is a back exercise, not an arm exercise," says Los Angeles-based certified trainer Keli Roberts, ACE spokesperson and Group Fitness Manager at Equinox in Pasadena, Calif. "It's very important to initiate the movement by pulling your shoulder blades down and back."

> Training this muscle also widens your back, making your waist appear smaller.

MISTAKES TO AVOID

➤ **Don't** lean backward by arching your back which can strain your back and cause you to rely on momentum and arm power rather than the strength of your lats.

➤ **Don't** hunch your back, round your shoulders or make your chest concave. These positions stress your entire upper body musculature and spine.

➤ **Don't** point your elbows backward instead of down to the floor. This inhibits full contraction of the lats.

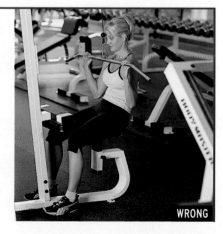

WRONG

A simple exercise for a strong back and beautiful, shapely shoulders.

THE RIGHT WAY

➤ Place your right hand and right knee on a bench with your back flat and head in line with your spine.

➤ Hold a dumbbell in your left hand with your arm hanging down directly in line with your shoulder, palm facing inward, elbow relaxed.

➤ Keeping your elbow close to your side, draw your shoulder blade toward your spine and pull your arm up and back from your shoulder. Concentrate on pulling with your back muscles, not your biceps.

➤ Keep your torso still. Don't rotate your hips and shoulders.

➤ Relax your muscles to return to the starting position, letting your shoulder blade slide forward and to the side as you slowly lower your arm toward the floor.

MUSCLES WORKED
latissimus dorsi , teres major, posterior deltoid

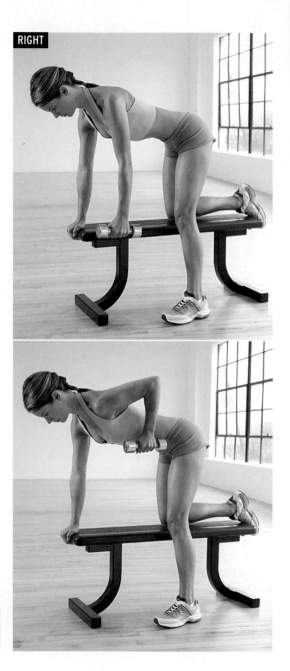

RIGHT

SINGLE-ARM LAT ROW

THE PAYOFF

The single-arm lat row develops and strengthens your rear shoulder and middle back muscles, training them as both movers and stabilizers. These muscles tend to respond quickly to training because they're generally under-developed. The overall effect will definitely be improved posture, as well as a sexy V-shape to your back and roundness to your shoulders.

WORKOUT GUIDELINES

Do 8 to 10 reps with each arm to complete one set, then repeat for 1 or 2 more sets. Use as much weight as you can to fatigue by 10 reps. To progress, increase your weight. Use 5 to 20 pounds.

EXPERT ADVICE

"Pre-contract your lat muscles before you lift the weight," says Mission Viejo, Calif.-based certified trainer Rob Glick, B.S., Exercise Science and Regional Group Fitness Director for Crunch Fitness. "This helps engage your back muscles to do all the work, not your biceps."

The effect will be improved posture, as well as a sexy V-shape to your back and roundness to your shoulders.

MISTAKES TO AVOID

➤ **Don't** sway your lower back. You'll have little to no support to lift the weight, and you may end up straining your back.

➤ **Don't** round your shoulders. It prevents the lats from doing the work, placing all the stress on your neck and upper back muscles.

➤ **Don't** rotate your shoulders or lift your elbow too high, as this takes the work away from the lats.

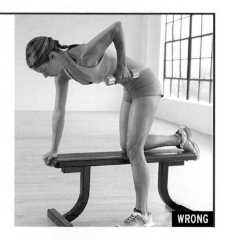

WRONG

Strengthen your upper body to maximize your exercise investment.

THE RIGHT WAY

➤ Lie faceup on a flat bench, with knees bent and heels on bench edge, holding a dumbbell over your chest with arms extended and elbows in a soft arc. Let the wide part of the dumbbell rest between your thumbs and index fingers.

➤ Keeping your head and hips on the bench, contract your abdominals, actively stabilizing your pelvis by bringing your spine to a neutral position and in contact with the bench.

➤ Slowly lower the dumbbell in an arc behind your head.

➤ Contract your lat muscles to bring the dumbbell back over your head to the starting position, keeping elbows in a slight arc. Repeat.

RIGHT

MUSCLES WORKED
latissimus dorsi, teres major, anterior deltoid, pectoralis major

DUMBBELL PULLOVER

THE PAYOFF
When it comes to efficient training, the pullover can optimize your effort. This versatile move develops sexy shoulder and back muscles. It simultaneously prevents injury by strengthening several large muscle groups at once, preparing the muscles of your chest, shoulders, middle back and upper arms for many activities and sports.

WORKOUT GUIDELINES
Do 2-3 sets of 8-12 reps, using as much weight as you can to fatigue by 12 reps. Rest 45-60 seconds between sets. To progress, do this exercise lying on a stability ball, which requires more balance. Use one 8- to 15-pound dumbbell.

EXPERT ADVICE
"If your shoulders are tight, you'll find it difficult to get your arms overhead comfortably without arching your back," says Tennessee-based physical therapist Debbie Ellison. "Accommodate tight shoulders by limiting your range of motion at first and stretch the front of your shoulders before attempting the pullover."

The pullover prevents injury by strengthening several large muscle groups at once.

MISTAKES TO AVOID
➤ **Don't** arch your back as you bring the dumbbell overhead. You will stress the lower-back muscles.
➤ **Don't** lower your arms too low behind your head. This strains the shoulder muscles and surrounding connective tissue.
➤ **Don't** tilt your head back, which can place stress on the cervical spine.

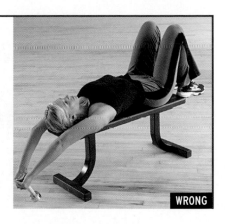

WRONG

In a slump? Strengthen your back extensors and carry yourself a little taller.

THE RIGHT WAY

➤ Lie facedown on the floor with your feet about hip-width apart, your arms by your sides. Contract your abs toward your spine so your abdomen is slightly off the floor.

➤ Lift your head, then your shoulders off the floor as you reach up and back with your arms, palms up. Raise arms up to shoulder height, pulling the shoulder blades to-gether and down. Then sweep arms out to the sides, palms down. Focus on maintaining the back extension and not lowering the torso. Hold for 4 counts.

➤ Raise your arms and torso slightly higher, then sweep your arms back to your sides. Lower the arms, torso and head sequentially to the starting position.

MUSCLES WORKED
erector spinae

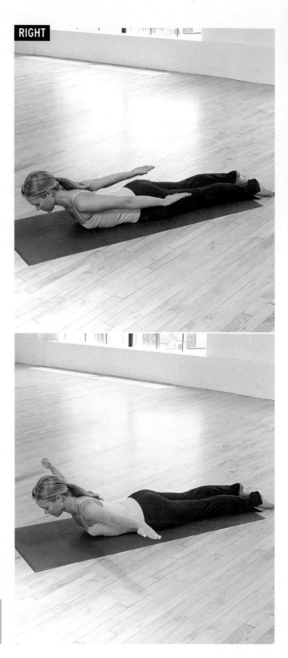

RIGHT

PRONE BACK EXTENSION

THE PAYOFF

You'll attain a stronger, healthier and more posture-perfect upper body by strengthening the muscles that extend along your entire spine. You'll also increase spine mobility and range of motion in your upper and middle back, which opens up the chest and front of the shoulders. Your muscles will be more limber and flexible overall, lowering your risk for back injury.

WORKOUT GUIDELINES

Do 6 reps, gradually working up to 12. When you can do 12 with good form, increase your range of motion so you can lift your upper body to about 30 degrees of extension (your chest will be up off the floor). To progress, do this movement with 2- to 3-pound dumbbells in each hand.

EXPERT ADVICE

"Contract your abdominals to limit excessive arching in the lower back region," says Karen Clippinger, M.S.P.E., a Los Angeles-based kinesiologist at UCLA. "Focus on strengthening the middle- and upper-back extensors, taking strain off your lower spine."

You'll attain a more posture-perfect upper body by strengthening the muscles that extend along your spine.

MISTAKES TO AVOID

➤ **Don't** let your lower back curve beyond its slight natural arch or you'll create pressure and tension in this area.

➤ **Don't** use jerky movements or excessive speed, which strain the delicate connective tissue of the spine as well as the back muscles.

➤ **Don't** let your belly sag or hyperextend your neck. Mistakes like these put pressure on your spine.

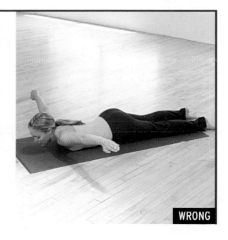

WRONG

Prevent injuries and get a shapely back with this effective exercise.

THE RIGHT WAY

➤ Hold a barbell with an overhand grip, arms straight, hands slightly wider than shoulder width apart. Stand with feet separated hip width, legs straight but not locked, bar hanging close to your thighs.

➤ Squeeze shoulder blades together to stabilize your spine and contract your abs. Then bend knees, hinging at hips and keeping back straight until back is approximately parallel to the floor and arms are extended, hanging just below knees.

➤ Maintain bentover position, keeping back muscles lengthened and head and neck in line with spine.

➤ Bend elbows, wrists straight, pulling bar up until nearly touching upper rib cage, then slowly lower. Straighten arms to start.

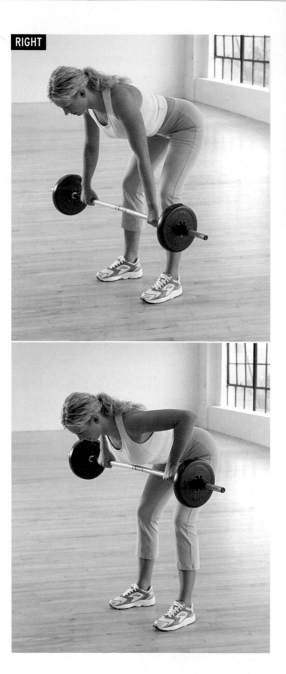

RIGHT

MUSCLES WORKED
latissimus dorsi, teres major, posterior deltoid, rhomboids, trapezius (lower fibers)

BENT-OVER BARBELL ROW

THE PAYOFF
Whether you're lifting a turkey out of the oven or boxes from a shelf, you need a strong torso to prevent back injuries. This exercise will help stabilize your torso by strengthening the muscles that are activated when bending, lifting and pulling. The bentover position requires sufficient back strength to maintain alignment as you lift and lower the barbell. You'll gain strength as well as a shapelier, sexier backside.

WORKOUT GUIDELINES
Do 2 to 3 sets of 8 to 12 reps, resting 45 to 60 seconds between sets. To learn proper form, practice with a light bar or stick first before adding weight. To progress, increase your weight. Use a 20- to 40-pound barbell.

EXPERT ADVICE
"As you pull the bar up, squeeze your shoulder blades together and down, and try not to round your upper back down to the bar," says certified strength specialist Jean Barrett Holloway, M.A. "Think about lifting your chest up and keeping your back tight; if you can't maintain your position, lighten the weight."

Whether you're lifting a turkey out of the oven or boxes from a shelf, you need a strong torso.

MISTAKES TO AVOID

➤ **Don't** lift your torso up as you lift the bar. This can place stress on your entire back.
➤ **Don't** drop your head, which can strain your neck and pull on the muscles of the upper back.
➤ **Don't** let your abs sag downward; this can cause you to lose torso stability and may also put pressure on your spine.

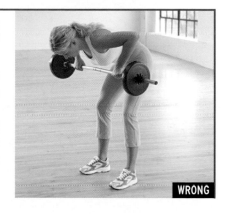

WRONG

BUTT & HAMSTRING EXERCISES

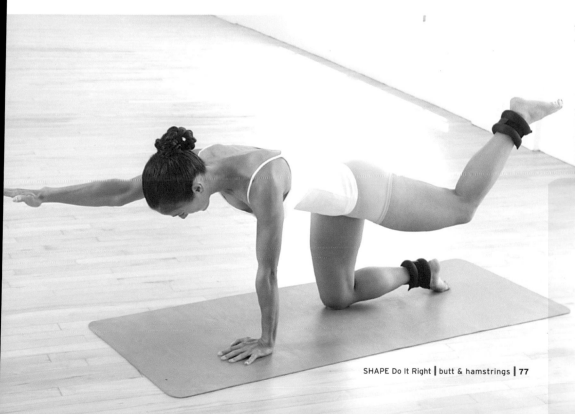

butt & hamstrings

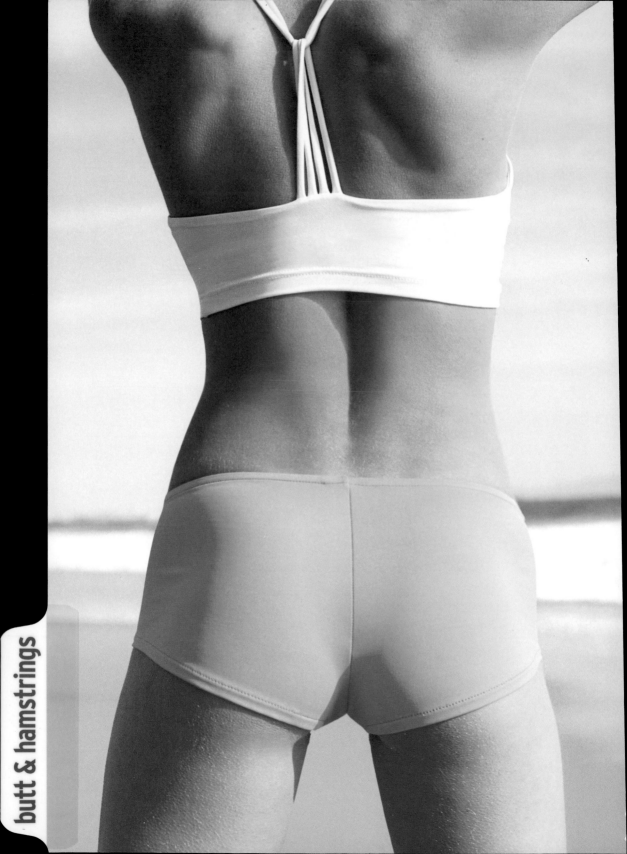

BUTT & HAMSTRINGS

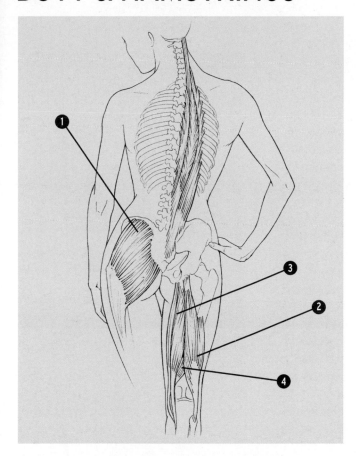

MUSCLES
1. gluteus maximus

hamstring group:
2. biceps femoris
3. semitendinosus
4. semimembranosus

The gluteus maximus is the largest and most superficial of the three gluteal muscles. The maximus originates on the outer edge of your pelvis, the bony structure at the base of your spine (sacrum) and lower part of your spine, then attaches to the rear thigh bone. The gluteus maximus is responsible for hip extension, lifting your leg behind you and rotating your thigh bone outward. The three hamstring muscles (biceps femoris, semimembranosus, semitendinosus) all attach to the "sit bones" at the base of your butt, running lengthwise on the rear of your thigh and attaching just below the knee on your lower leg bones. They work with the gluteus maximus during hip extension and are independently responsible for flexing your knees. Both of these muscle groups also work with the quadriceps, hip abductors and adductors for multi-muscle exercises.

Borrow this move from ballet for beautiful buns and toned inner thighs.

THE RIGHT WAY

➤ Stand with your feet slightly wider than shoulder-width apart, knees straight (not locked), abdominals in and tailbone pointing toward the floor. Hold 5-pound dumbbells with palms facing your thighs.

➤ Shift your weight to your heels and rotate your feet and legs out from your hips as a unit, so that your knees and feet point toward the sides. Don't let your feet turn out past your knees. Shift your weight forward so that it's evenly distributed over the length of your feet.

➤ Slowly bend your knees and lower your body as far as you can, keeping your weight evenly distributed and your heels on the floor. Do not lower further than the point at which thighs are parallel to the floor. Slowly straighten knees (don't hyperextend them) and raise your body to the starting position.

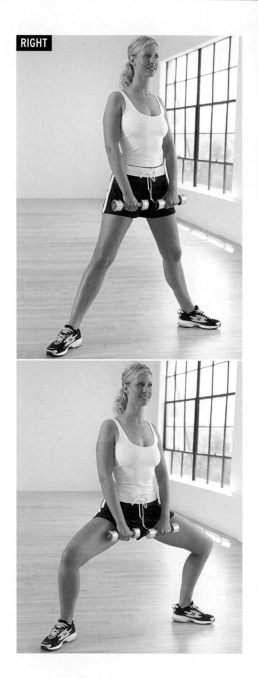

RIGHT

MUSCLES WORKED
gluteus maximus, hamstrings, quadriceps, hip adductors

PLIÉ WITH DUMBBELLS

THE PAYOFF

It's no secret that most of us would like to have toned buns and inner thighs. The real secret is finding a great exercise to get this job done. Dancers have known of one for ages, and we're blowing the lid off of it. The turned-out second-position plié is a variation on the common strength-training squat. The turned-out stance targets the inner thighs.

WORKOUT GUIDELINES

Do 2 to 3 sets of 10 to 12 repetitions, resting 45 to 60 seconds between sets. To progress, increase your weight and also try to increase your range of motion. Use 8- to 15-pound dumbbells in each hand.

EXPERT ADVICE

"As you plié, focus on the tailbone moving straight up and straight down as if pointing downward like an arrow at the floor," says Karen Clippinger, M.S.P.E, a Los Angeles-based kinesiologist and instructor at UCLA. "This helps to emphasize the buttocks and the inner thigh muscles, along with maintaining precision technique."

The turned-out second-position plié is a variation on the common strength-training squat.

MISTAKES TO AVOID

➤ **Don't** let your knees roll inward of your feet, which stresses both the knee and ankle joints as well as the surrounding ligaments and tendons.

➤ **Don't** drop your hips so low that your pelvis changes alignment and your back arches. This causes tension in your lower back.

➤ **Don't** lock your knees as you straighten your legs, which may cause knee and back stress.

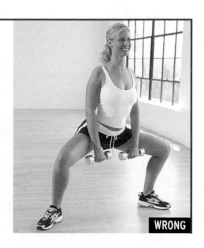

WRONG

Toned hamstrings make thighs sexier and improve your posture.

THE RIGHT WAY

➤ Lie facedown on the machine so your hips line up with the bend of the pad. (If your machine is flat, place a rolled towel underneath your hips for lower-back support.) Adjust the ankle pad so it's resting on the back of your ankles and your kneecaps are off the machine pad.

➤ Grasp the handles and pull your navel toward your spine to activate your abs. Tighten your buttocks and lift your thighs slightly off the machine while keeping your hipbones in contact with pad.

➤ Keeping buttocks contracted, slowly bend your knees, bringing your heels toward – but not all the way to – your butt. Stop when your heels have passed your

knees. Hold for a moment and then slowly return your heels to the starting position, straightening but not locking your knees.

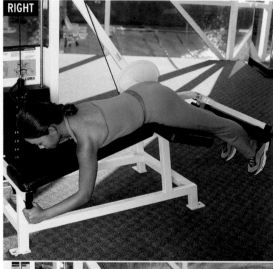

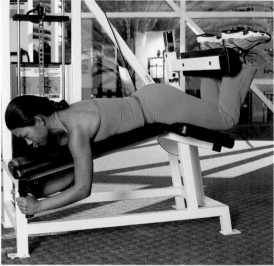

MUSCLES WORKED
hamstrings, gluteus maximus

PRONE HAMSTRING CURL

THE PAYOFF
This classic hamstring exercise gives a sexy, athletic curve to your rear thigh. Strong hamstrings – important for running, hiking and cycling – also help protect your knees from injury and promote good posture by working your abdominals to balance your pelvis, resulting in a stabilized, neutral position.

WORKOUT GUIDELINES
Start with 1 or 2 sets of 15 reps. Begin with 30-60 pounds (depending on the machine).

When you can do 15 reps comfortably, increase the weight and drop to 8-10 reps, gradually working back up to 15 reps.

EXPERT ADVICE
"The key to doing this exercise correctly is contracting your butt and slightly lifting your thighs off the pad," says Los Angeles trainer Keli Roberts. "When your glutes are contracted, it's impossible to arch your back. Concentrate on maintaining this position throughout the entire set."

Strong hamstrings promote good posture by working your abdominals to balance your pelvis, resulting in a stabilized, natural position.

MISTAKES TO AVOID
➤ **Don't** arch your back or stick up your butt. Not only will your hamstring work be less efficient, but this can also be stressful to your back.
➤ **Don't** adjust the ankle pad so that it's resting on your heels instead of your ankles; this will place stress on your knees when you perform the move.
➤ **Don't** make the alternative mistake of adjusting the ankle pad so it sits on your calves. This limits the range of motion.

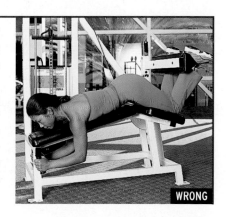

WRONG

Boost your rear view with the easy-to-do chair bridge.

butt & hamstrings

THE RIGHT WAY

➤ Lie on your back on the floor with your knees bent (less than 90 degrees) and your heels on the seat of a chair. Relax your arms by your sides.

➤ Contract your abdominal muscles to bring your pubic bone toward your waist. Then, pressing down on the chair seat with your heels, take four seconds to lift your pelvis, then your waist and upper back, off the floor to form a straight line from your knees to your shoulders. Hold this position for four seconds, concentrating on pressing the tops of the thighs farther upward without overarching your back.

➤ Take four more seconds to return to the starting position, lowering the back, then the waist and pelvis.

MUSCLES WORKED
hamstrings, gluteus maximus

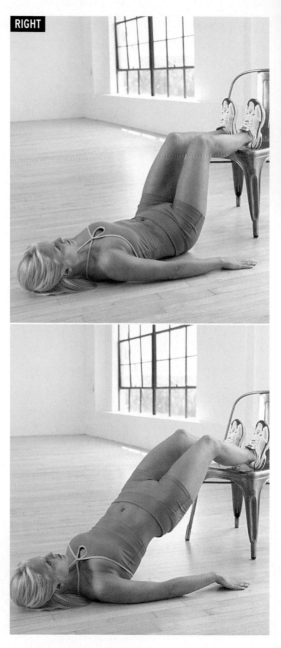

RIGHT

CHAIR BRIDGE

THE PAYOFF

While strengthening and toning the gluteus maximus and hamstring muscles, this easy-to-do exercise mimics a movement pattern that promotes strong posture for all sorts of basic activities, including walking and running.

WORKOUT GUIDELINES

Do 8 reps, eventually working up to 12, as part of your lower-body routine. When you can do 12 reps with good form, progress to doing the move with one leg extended. For an even greater challenge, attach a 3-pound ankle weight to the extended leg. (Gradually increase the weight up to no more than 10 pounds.)

EXPERT ADVICE

"Keep your upper body relaxed and rib cage flattened as you lift and lower the torso," says Karen Clippinger, M.S.P.E, Los Angeles-based kinesiologist and instructor at UCLA. "This places the focus on your pelvis and forces your buttocks and hamstrings to initiate the movement as opposed to straining with your neck, shoulders and arms."

This exercise mimics a movement pattern that promotes strong posture for all sorts of basic activities.

MISTAKES TO AVOID

➤ **Don't** lift hips so high that you arch your back and press out your rib cage. This places stress on the lower-back muscles and ligaments.

➤ **Don't** press down with your hands and arms to assist the lift; this lessens the effectiveness of the exercise and takes work away from your buttocks and hamstrings.

➤ **Don't** tuck your pelvis under to start. You'll decrease the range of motion and force your spine out of a neutral position.

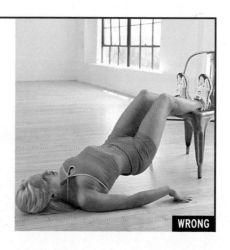

WRONG

One great move to reshape the backs of your thighs.

THE RIGHT WAY

➤ Stand facing an upright support, such as a pole or wall, with a 2-pound ankle weight attached to your right ankle. Lean slightly forward with your torso, resting your forearms against the support so your elbows are just about shoulder height.

➤ Keeping your weight over your slightly bent left leg, extend your right leg behind you, resting the toes of your right foot on the floor.

➤ Slightly bend your right leg, then take three seconds to slowly raise the whole leg toward the ceiling until your thigh creates a straight line with your torso and hips. Pause briefly, then take four seconds to lower the leg to the floor.

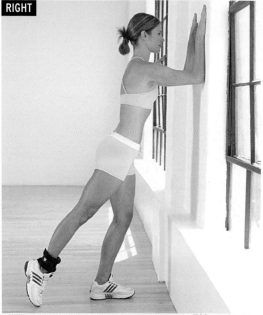

RIGHT

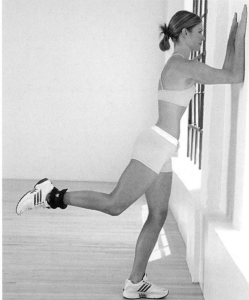

MUSCLES WORKED

Hamstrings group: semimembranosus, semitendinosus, biceps femoris; gluteus maximus

STANDING HAMSTRING CURL

THE PAYOFF

The standing hamstring curl is one of the best ways to add strong curves to your thighs. This move strengthens the often-neglected hamstring muscles. Toning this muscle group will add contour and definition to the backs of your thighs. In addition to their key role in basic movements like walking and running, strong hamstrings promote healthy posture and reduce your risk of injury.

WORKOUT GUIDELINES

Do 8 reps, then switch legs (and the weight) and repeat on the opposite leg. Work up to performing 12 reps on each leg. As you get stronger, or to increase the intensity, move the supporting leg farther back from the wall.

EXPERT ADVICE

"To utilize more hamstrings than buttocks for this exercise, bend your heel up toward the buttocks of the working leg before you even lift your leg," says Karen Clippinger, Los-Angeles based kinesiologist and instructor at UCLA. "By pre-contracting your hamstrings, you'll ensure that your hamstrings will do most of the lifting."

The standing hamstring curl strengthens the hamstring muscles to add definition to the backs of your thighs.

MISTAKES TO AVOID

➤ **Don't** lift your working leg so high that your back arches. This will cause you to strain your lower back to compensate for the arch.

➤ **Don't** use momentum to lift your working leg, especially with an ankle weight on. This can put stress on the knee and hip joints.

➤ **Don't** stand with your support knee straight or locked. Keep it slightly bent to prevent hyperextension of the knee and lower back.

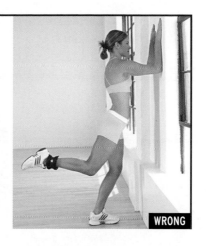

WRONG

Behind every great bottom is a perfect squat.

THE RIGHT WAY

➤ Stand with feet slightly more than hip-width apart, toes out slightly, knees aligned with midfoot. Hold dumbbells at your sides, palms in.

➤ Keeping your pelvis in neutral position, expand your chest and lift your rib cage. Inhale, hold your breath briefly and draw the lower part of your abs toward your spine.

➤ Maintaining this posture, look straight ahead and lower your body as if sitting back in a chair, keeping heels on the floor and pressure evenly distributed through your feet. (Your torso will lean forward slightly.) Lower until thighs are as close to parallel to floor as possible.

➤ Drive back up (exhaling when past the most difficult point) to starting position, keeping heels on the floor.

RIGHT

MUSCLES WORKED
gluteus maximus, hamstrings, quadriceps

THE PAYOFF

This mother of all lower-body exercises strengthens and firms your glutes, quadriceps and hamstrings all at once. It also calls upon your inner-thigh and outer-hip muscles to stabilize your pelvis and knees, their primary function in everyday activities such as bending and squatting.

WORKOUT GUIDELINES

Start with 1-2 sets of 12-15 reps, resting 45 to 60 seconds between sets. Choose a weight that causes you to fatigue at 12-15 reps, whether it be 5- or 20-pound dumbbells. To progress, gradually work up to 2-3 sets and increase your weight enough to fatigue in only 10-12 reps per set.

EXPERT ADVICE

"The lowering phase is where you get the biggest bang for your butt," says Mark Cibrario, owner of The Trainer's Club, a private studio in Northbrook, Ill. "Take a full 3-4 seconds to sink down through your hips." Pause at the bottom of the movement, then drive up, using your butt and legs to stand.

This mother of all lower-body exercises strengthens and firms your glutes, quadriceps and hamstrings.

MISTAKES TO AVOID

➤ **Don't** let your knees roll inward or bow outward; this causes excessive joint stress.

➤ **Don't** let your knees shoot out over your toes; this can damage tendons and cartilage.

➤ **Don't** round your back; this can cause back injury. Don't squat lower than the point at which your thighs are parallel to the floor or at which you maintain control of your neutral spine.

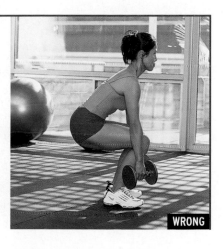

WRONG

Need a lift? Try one of the most simple and effective lower-body moves.

THE RIGHT WAY

➤ Stand, holding dumbbells, arms hanging by your sides, palms facing each other. (Harder version: With elbows bent, hold dumbbells on your shoulders.) Place your feet hip-width apart, tighten your abs and look straight ahead.

➤ Keeping your abs tight and chest up, take an exaggerated step forward with your right foot so your right knee and ankle line up. Left knee is bent and approaching the floor, heel is lifted. Distribute your weight evenly between your feet.

➤ Lower your body until your left knee is a few inches from the ground, then push back up to the starting position. Do recommended number of reps, then switch legs and repeat.

MUSCLES WORKED
gluteus maximus, hamstrings, quadriceps, gastrocnemius, soleus

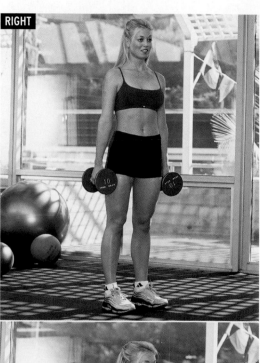

RIGHT

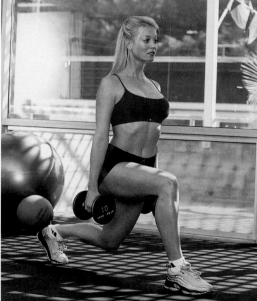

LUNGE

THE PAYOFF

No exercise firms and strengthens your lower body – especially your butt, quadriceps, hamstrings and calves – more effectively than the lunge. Lunges recruit muscles in compound ways, taking your body through motions you do in every-day activities, and helping you to maintain your balance.

WORKOUT GUIDELINES

Do 3 alternating sets of 10-15 reps on each leg, starting with no weight if necessary, working up to a 20-pound dumbbell in each hand. Master your form before adding weight. To progress, increase weight or lunge with the rear leg kept straight.

EXPERT ADVICE

"The lunge is an exaggerated move that requires a lot of balance," says Juan Carlos Santana, M.S., C.S.C.S., director of the Institute of Human Performance in Boca Raton, Fla. "If necessary, steady yourself by resting one hand lightly on the back of a chair to help you perfect your form."

Lunges recruit muscles in compound ways, taking your body through motions you do in everyday activities.

MISTAKES TO AVOID

➤ **Don't** step across; it's important to step straight forward, feet hip-width apart, to maintain balance.

➤ **Don't** step meekly forward: You may lose your balance and your rear leg won't "work" as much.

➤ **Don't** look down; focusing straight ahead will help keep your body properly aligned. Think vertical, not horizontal: Move hips up and down, not forward and back.

➤ **Don't** shift your weight forward; keep it over your hips to prevent excess pressure on your knee.

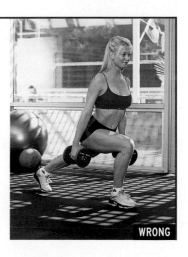

WRONG

Update a traditional back leg lift and you'll get all-around benefits.

THE RIGHT WAY

➤ On a soft surface, get on your hands and knees with spine in a neutral position and head in line with spine.

➤ Wearing a 3-pound weight around each ankle, slide left knee back along the floor until leg is almost straight.

➤ Slowly raise leg until thigh is parallel to the floor. (To target hamstrings more effectively, keep knee slightly bent and lift from your knee, not buttocks.)

➤ Raise your right arm forward, even with your shoulder. Pause and slowly return to the starting position, bringing your arm back down first.

➤ Throughout the exercise, contract your abs to keep your back from overarching and keep your pelvis and chest facing squarely toward the floor.

MUSCLES WORKED
hamstrings, gluteus maximus, trapezius,
erector spinae, anterior deltoid

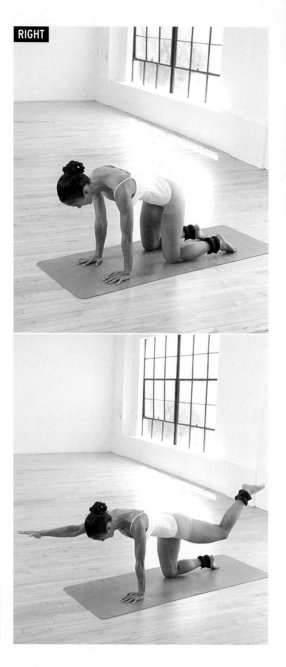

RIGHT

BACK LEG LIFT

THE PAYOFF
This move is a safe and excellent way to strengthen and tone the backs of your thighs, buttocks and even your back and shoulders. You will target your hamstrings, muscles that tend to be low in strength and prone to injury. When you add a front arm raise to the move, you'll challenge your balance and coordination, stabilize your torso and work your upper body and back.

WORKOUT GUIDELINES
Do 8 reps on each side, working up to 12. When your strength and bal-ance increase, add a 1-pound dumbbell to the arm lift. In 1-pound increments, gradually increase ankle resistance from 3 to 10 pounds and arm resistance from 1 to 3 pounds.

EXPERT ADVICE
"Move slowly and concentrate on lengthening your leg as you slide it along the floor, knee bent, before you lift," says Karen Clippinger, Los Angeles-based kinesiologist and instructor at UCLA. "This en-gages your hamstrings more ef-fectively to perform the movement rather than using your buttocks."

You will target your hamstrings, muscles that tend to be low in strength and prone to injury.

MISTAKES TO AVOID
➤ **Don't** lift your leg so high that you arch your lower back. This places stress on your back muscles and your spine.
➤ **Don't** "throw" your lifting leg upward; this can also stress your spine.
➤ **Don't** sink into your shoulder blades, round your back or sag your belly. You'll de-stabilize your torso, giving you very little support to perform the movement.

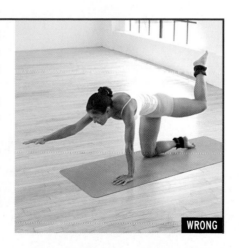
WRONG

One effective move for firming and strengthening your butt, hips and thighs.

THE RIGHT WAY

➤ Lie facedown and backward on either an angled or horizontal hyperextension bench with hip crease at bench edge, head pointing toward roller pad and legs hanging toward floor (depending on height of machine, your toes may touch the ground).

➤ Hold the roller pad with your hands shoulder-width apart — or for more stability, place your forearms, hands clasped, on the pad.

➤ Separate legs in a V, feet hip-width apart, and contract your abdominals to keep spine naturally curved and take tension off lower back.

➤ Squeeze your shoulder blades down and together, stabilizing the position so you're not tensing your shoulders or hands.

➤ Without moving

torso, but keeping legs straight, contract buttocks, lifting legs up to hip height; use inner thighs to bring legs together at top of movement.

➤ Slowly lower legs, separating them into a V at bottom of movement.

RIGHT

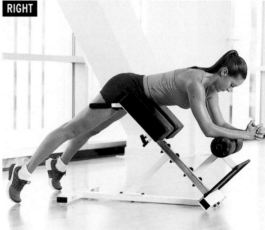

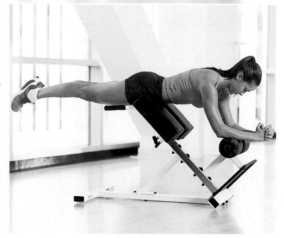

MUSCLES WORKED
gluteus maximus, upper fibers of the hamstrings, gluteus minimus, adductors

HANGING DOUBLE-LEG LIFT

THE PAYOFF
This move perfectly isolates your butt, the upper fibers of your hamstrings and your inner-thigh muscles, since you use your abdominal, lower-back and scapular muscles to stabilize your torso against the bench. You'll quickly achieve an incredibly strong and sculpted lower body that will carry you through almost any activity.

WORKOUT GUIDELINES
Do this move as part of a regular lower-body strength program. Using no added weight, do 2-3 sets of 8-12 reps each, resting 30-60 seconds between sets. To progress, attach 2- to 5-pound weights to each ankle (as long as you feel no added stress on your lower back).

EXPERT ADVICE
"Instead of using your back to facilitate lifting your legs, 'pre-contract' your abdominal and buttocks muscles," says Karen Andes, Philadelphia-based teacher, trainer and author of *A Woman's Book of Strength* (Perigee, 1995). "Also, begin by taking a moment to visualize the buttocks doing the work."

Contract your abdominals to keep the spine naturally curved and take tension off the lower back.

MISTAKES TO AVOID

➤ **Don't** swing your legs upward, letting momentum take over; this can injure the lower back.

➤ **Don't** let your abdominal muscles sag against the bench; this can cause torso instability and impede your ability to raise your legs high enough.

➤ **Don't** lift your head; this over-stresses the neck muscles and takes the spine out of alignment.

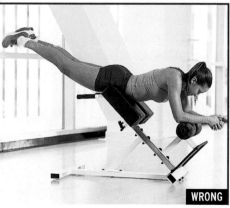

WRONG

Get gravity-defying glutes and toned legs in one move.

THE RIGHT WAY

➤ Attach an ankle strap to a low-cable pulley machine, then adjust an incline bench to 45 degrees and place it approximately a foot behind and just to the left of the cable pulley.

➤ With ankle strap around your right ankle, lean the front of your body against the back of the incline bench with your left knee on the seat and your right leg slightly bent, hanging down to the side and just ahead of the bench.

➤ Contract abdominals, bringing spine to a neutral position and pressing the front of your left hip and thigh firmly against the back of the bench.

➤ Maintaining this position, contract your buttocks and sweep your right leg behind you, lifting it only as high as you can while keeping your left hipbone against the bench.

➤ Pause, squeezing buttocks at the top of the movement, then bring leg back to starting position. Repeat for all reps, then switch legs.

RIGHT

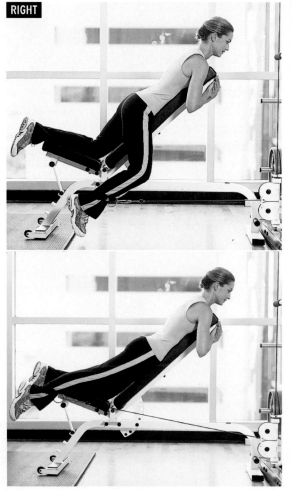

MUSCLES WORKED
gluteus maximus, upper fibers of the hamstrings

INCLINE CABLE HIP EXTENSION

THE PAYOFF
Because your entire body is stabilized on an incline bench, this move really hones your buttocks and upper hamstring muscles, working them through their fullest range of motion and allowing you to use more weight to get the final squeeze (something that you can't always get while standing). It also keeps your spine in alignment, which will assist in preventing injury as well as helping to perfect your technique.

WORKOUT GUIDELINES
Starting with 15-20 pounds, do 2-3 sets of 10-15 reps on each side, resting 30-60 seconds between sets. Increase weight in 2½-pound increments as you progress.

EXPERT ADVICE
"Draw the leg straight back as if circumscribing a semicircle," says Jon Giswold, New York City-based trainer and author of *Basic Training* (St. Martin's Press, 1998). "Moving in this way will help you fully utilize all the muscle fibers in your buttocks and hamstrings muscles."

This move really hones your buttocks and upper hamstring muscles.

MISTAKES TO AVOID

➤ **Don't** allow your hipbone to lift from the back of the bench; this can destabilize your body, resulting in the use of momentum rather than promoting muscle work.
➤ **Don't** use too much weight; doing so can place stress on your spine.
➤ **Don't** place the incline bench too far from the low-cable-pulley machine; this can impede proper alignment.

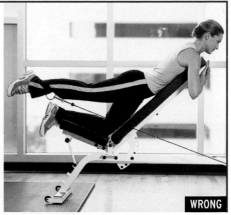

WRONG

Sculpt a stronger lower body with one powerful move.

butt & hamstrings

THE RIGHT WAY

➤ Place a straight barbell just over insteps, and stand with feet on a pair of weight plates (so heels are on floor), just about hip-width apart.

➤ Keeping back straight, bend knees slightly while hinging forward at hips to grasp bar with an overhand grip, hands slightly wider than hips, and raise bar to start position at knee height.

➤ Driving from your legs, with eyes focused ahead and back straight, lift torso so bar passes knees; continue extending hips and straighten until you're standing erect with bar at thighs.

➤ Bend knees and lower bar to starting position, keeping back straight and shoulders relaxed.

MUSCLES WORKED
gluteus maximus, hamstrings, erector spinae

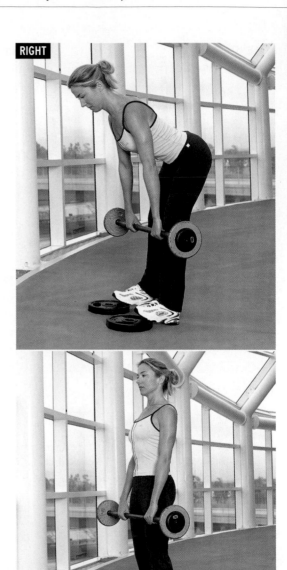

RIGHT

BENT-LEGGED DEAD LIFT

THE PAYOFF
This move works that curvaceous area below your waist – lower back, glutes and hamstrings – yielding a more beautifully sculpted lower body. Your stronger, sexier hips and thighs will power you through all kinds of high-endurance activities, especially sports that involve lots of running and jumping.

WORKOUT GUIDELINES
Do 2-3 sets of 10-12 reps, lifting 20-50 pounds. Rest 60 seconds between sets. When you can complete all reps with good form, increase the weight.

EXPERT ADVICE
"Always initiate this lift with your leg muscles, not your back," says Juan Carlos Santana, M.S., C.S.C.S., director of Optimum Performance Systems in Boca Raton, Fla., "And don't straighten your legs until the bar has reached your thighs."

This move works that curvaceous area below your waist, yielding a more beautifully sculpted lower body.

MISTAKES TO AVOID
➤ **Don't** round your back. You'll lose stability in your torso, which could injure your back.
➤ **Don't** start with the bar too far from your body. Otherwise, you may not allow your leg muscles to do the work, also potentially harming your back.
➤ **Don't** overcompensate for weakness in your legs by arching your back as you stand. This will only end up stressing your lower back.

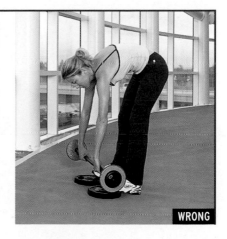

WRONG

Here's one foolproof move for a stronger, shapelier lower body.

THE RIGHT WAY

➤ Stand on your left foot, holding a dumbbell in each hand with arms hanging by your sides, palms facing in.

➤ Lift your right knee up to about hip level so that your right heel hangs in line with your right knee, torso erect, shoulders in line with hips, hips squared.

➤ Squeeze shoulder blades down and together, stabilizing torso, then contract your abdominals throughout the entire exercise as you sit back into your left heel, bending your left knee and lowering your hips as much as you can while staying balanced, torso erect.

➤ Straighten your left knee as you contract buttocks to press up to starting position.

➤ Repeat for all reps; switch legs.

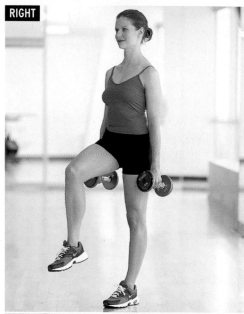

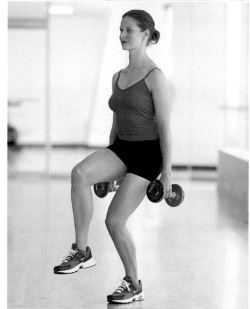

RIGHT

MUSCLES WORKED
gluteus maximus, hamstrings, quadriceps

ONE-LEGGED SQUAT

THE PAYOFF

Thanks to the one-legged challenge to your balance, this move forces all of your lower-body muscles – plus your abs – to work harder for better, quicker results. One leg is usually stronger than the other, so working them independently increases muscle stimulation in each leg, balancing the strength ratio from side to side.

WORKOUT GUIDELINES

Starting with 5- to 10-pound dumbbells, do 2-3 sets of 10-15 reps with each leg (complete reps on both legs for 1 set). Progress by keeping the lifted leg straight as you squat.

EXPERT ADVICE

"Lift your toes slightly inside your standing shoe, which automatically shifts your body weight back toward your heel," says Jon Giswold, New York City-based trainer and author of *Basic Training* (St. Martin's Press, 1998). "This ensures that you target your buttocks and hamstrings and don't stress your knee."

This move forces all of your lower-body muscles – plus your abs – to work harder for better, quicker results.

MISTAKES TO AVOID

➤ **Don't** round your upper back as you squat; this causes the torso to collapse forward and abs to relax, leaving little torso support.

➤ **Don't** let your standing knee travel in front of your standing toes. This can place stress on knee ligaments and tendons, and also destabilize the knee.

➤ **Don't** lean back into the squat; this can put excess strain and pressure on your lower spine, and you also may lose your balance.

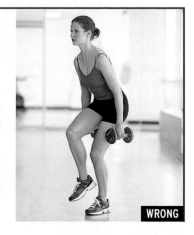

WRONG

An incredibly precise move for leaner legs and a toned tush.

THE RIGHT WAY

➤ Lying faceup on floor with arms relaxed at your sides, place heels in the center of a stability ball, legs straight and feet slightly less than hip-width apart (the closer your feet, the more challenging the move).

➤ Contract your abdominals to stabilize back, hips and pelvis.

➤ Lift your hips up off floor into a bridge so your body forms one straight line from your shoulders to your ankles; at the same time, roll the stability ball toward your hips by bending your knees and pulling the ball with your heels.

➤ Be sure to shift your weight only onto your shoulders (not into your neck).

➤ Pause at the top of the lift, then roll the stability ball back out by pushing it away with your heels until your legs are straight, keeping your hips raised in bridge position.

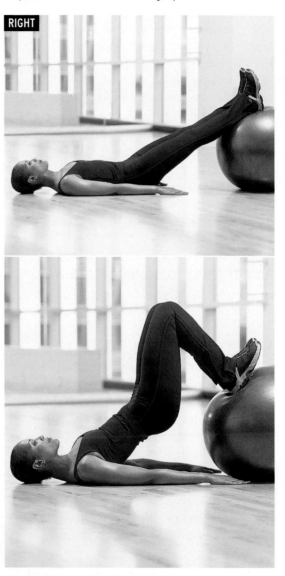

RIGHT

MUSCLES WORKED
hamstrings, gluteus maximus

BALL-BRIDGE HAMSTRING CURL

THE PAYOFF
No exercise is better at isolating your hamstrings and boosting your buns, thanks to the added resistance you get from rolling the ball. The ball-bridge hamstring curl also develops core strength and pelvis stability, which translates to better posture and the ability to maintain neutral spinal alignment. Finally, this move stretches tight hip flexors, making you more coordinated and agile in sports and daily activities.

WORKOUT GUIDELINES
Begin with 2 sets of 10-15 reps, resting 1 minute between sets. When this is no longer challenging, add a third set.

EXPERT ADVICE
"Keep even tension on the ball by pressing down with your heels, and focus on dragging the ball toward your hips in a straight line," says Leigh Crews, NASM, The Cooper Institute-certified trainer and owner of Dynalife Fitness Inc. in Rome, Ga. "This will ensure that you're working the hamstrings, not the quadriceps, and that neither leg is dominating the effort of the movement."

No exercise is better at isolating your hamstrings and boosting your buns.

MISTAKES TO AVOID
➤ **Don't** arch your back as you roll the ball underneath you; this can put pressure on your lower back and spine.
➤ **Don't** let your knees open out to the sides so they're not in line with your ankles; this places stress on the knee tendons and hip rotators.
➤ **Don't** place entire foot on the ball as you roll it toward your hips; this can stress the knee tendons and ligaments as well as pull on your shin muscles.

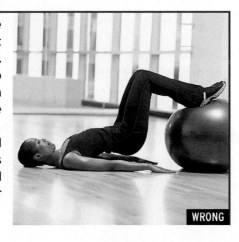

WRONG

CHEST EXERCISES

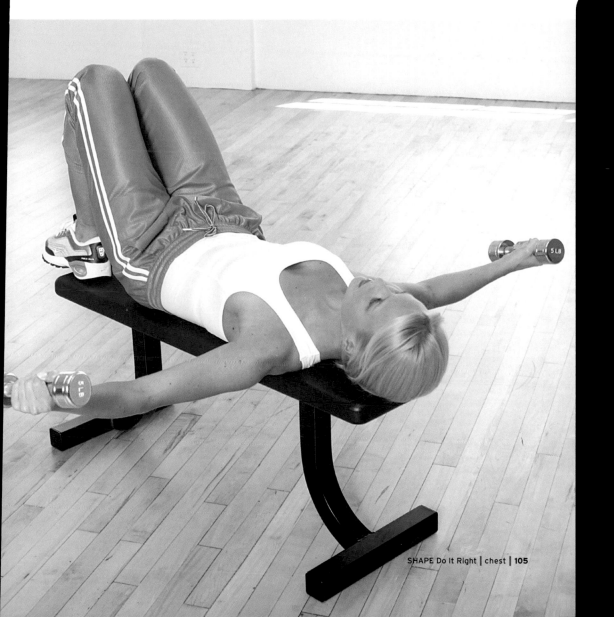

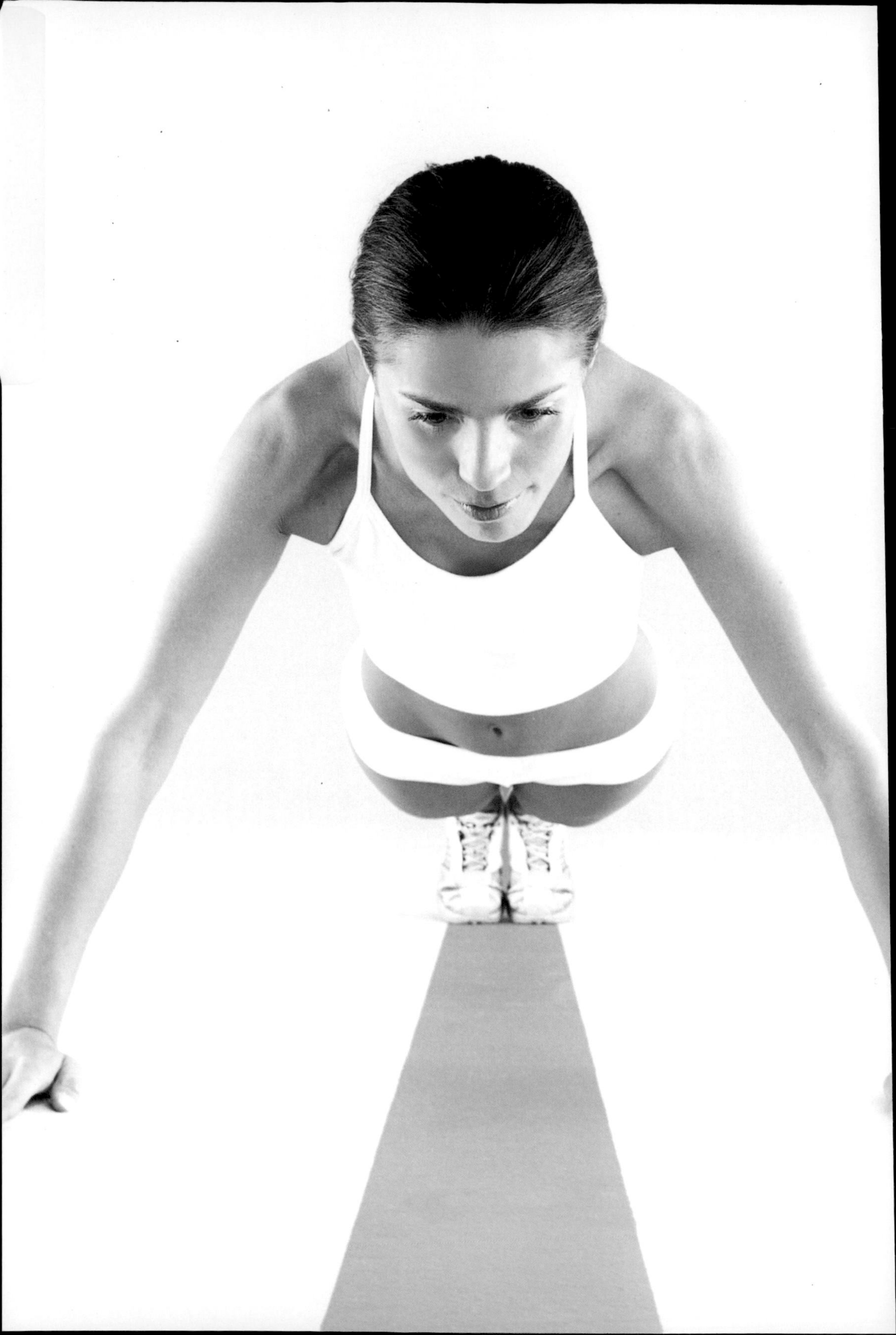

CHEST

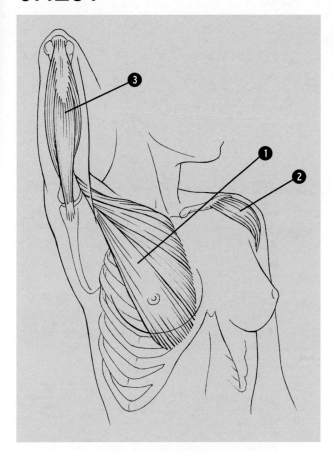

MUSCLES
1. pectoralis major
2. anterior deltoid
3. triceps

Your main chest muscle, the pectoralis major, is a large fan-shaped muscle with multiple attachments. One portion attaches to the middle and inner part of your collarbone, working with the anterior deltoid (your front shoulder muscle) to move your arms forward, upward and rotate the arm inward. The other part attaches on your breastbone (sternum) and upper six ribs, and is stimulated only in downward and forward arm movements. Both portions attach together near the top of your upper arm bone. The serratus anterior, located on either side of your rib cage, and the pectoralis minor, a small muscle under the pectoralis major, stabilize your shoulder blades as your arms move forward. In addition, the triceps is involved in any chest pushing motion.

Give yourself a lift — and tone your shoulders and triceps, too — with this one move.

THE RIGHT WAY

➤ Sit on a flat bench with dumbbells resting vertically on your thighs, knees bent and feet flat on the floor.

➤ Roll back, "kicking" the dumbbells up over your chest, to lie on the bench (contract abs so your back touches the bench); put heels on the bench's edge.

➤ Press the dumbbells directly above your chest, palms forward, arms straight (not locked), dumbbells almost touching.

➤ Slowly bend elbows, lowering the weights down and out toward the sides of your chest. Stop when your arms form a 90-degree angle, upper arms in line with shoulders.

➤ Slowly press arms back up to starting position without locking elbows.

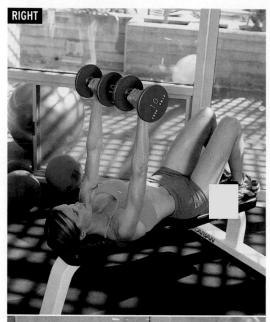

RIGHT

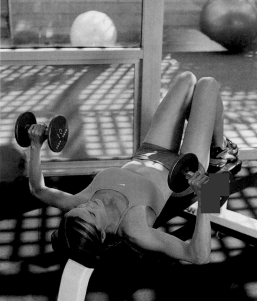

MUSCLES WORKED
pectoralis major, anterior deltoid, triceps

DUMBBELL CHEST PRESS

THE PAYOFF

The dumbbell chest press firms and strengthens your chest, shoulders and even the backs of your arms. It's an even more functional chest exercise than the barbell bench press, since working your arms independently uses more of your smaller stabilizing muscles.

WORKOUT GUIDELINES

Start with 1 to 3 sets of 8 to 10 reps, resting 45 to 60 seconds between each set. Use enough weight to fatigue by the 10th rep. Progress by increasing weight when 10 reps is no longer challenging. Use a 5- to 20-pound dumbbell in each hand.

EXPERT ADVICE

"To promote fluidity and consistency, pinpoint a spot on the ceiling directly above your chest and press the dumbbells to that point for each repetition," says Los Angeles-based certified trainer Keli Roberts, ACE spokesperson and Group Fitness Manager at Equinox in Pasadena, Calif. "This simple technique will dramatically improve the quality of your press."

The dumbbell chest press firms and strengthens your chest, shoulders and the backs of your arms.

MISTAKES TO AVOID

➤ **Don't** lower your elbows too far. This will put your shoulders at greater risk for injury.
➤ **Don't** arch your back or push with your feet to hoist the dumbbells. This places extra stress on your back.
➤ **Don't** bend your wrists; to protect them, position them so that they're in line with your forearms and elbows.

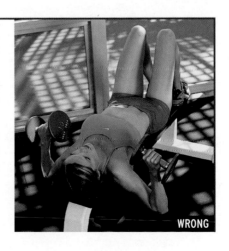

WRONG

A chest-and-shoulder shaper that really works.

chest

THE RIGHT WAY

➤ Lie on your back on a bench with head on one end of the bench, knees bent and heels on the bench's edge. Hold a dumbbell in each hand, and raise arms upward, directly above chest, palms facing in, about one inch apart. Keep arms, wrists and elbows slightly rounded. Arms are in line with shoulders.

➤ Slowly lower arms in an arc-like pattern until you feel a gentle stretch across the front of your shoulders (until your elbows are even with shoulder height).

➤ Pause, then slowly raise arms to the starting position. Be sure to maintain control throughout the movement, not relying on speed or momentum to raise or lower the weight.

MUSCLES WORKED
pectoralis major, anterior deltoid

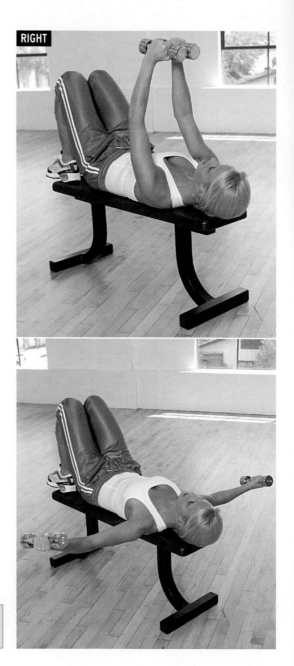

RIGHT

PEC FLY

THE PAYOFF

This is a great exercise for toning the muscles of the chest and shoulders. A strong chest can help give a little lift to the bust area, and strong shoulders help you look better in sleeveless tops. But it's not all about aesthetics: A strong chest and shoulders come in handy whenever you need your arms to cross your body, such as when hitting forehand in tennis or picking up a child.

WORKOUT GUIDELINES

Do 1–3 sets of 8 reps, working up to sets of 12 reps each. Rest 60 seconds between sets. To progress, gradually increase the resistance in 1- to 2-pound increments, to as much as 15 pounds per hand. Each time you increase the weight, begin with 8 reps per set, working back up to 12 reps per set before the next weight increase. Use 5 to 15 pounds in each hand.

EXPERT ADVICE:

"Think of wrapping your arms around a barrel to help maintain the arc shape ," says Karen Clippinger, M.S.P.E, a Los Angeles-based kinesiologist and instructor at UCLA. "This will help you isolate your chest muscles instead of using your arms."

A strong chest and shoulders come in handy whenever you need your arms to cross your body.

MISTAKES TO AVOID

➤ **Don't** perform this exercise too quickly. Rushing through the movement can cause elbows and wrists to hyperextend.
➤ **Don't** lower your arms below shoulder height, which can stress the shoulder joint as well as the delicate connective tissue.
➤ **Don't** let your lower back arch as you lower your arms. This places undue tension on the spine.

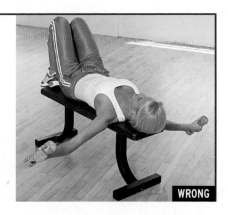
WRONG

Lift and improve the overall appearance of your chest with one great move.

THE RIGHT WAY

➤ Adjust an incline bench to a 30-degree angle; position the bench equally between two single-handle low cables. Set the weight, then sit on the bench and grasp the cable handles, putting your knuckles together and keeping elbows slightly bent.

➤ Lie back, with your knees bent and your feet on the edge of the bench. Holding the cable handles with your knuckles barely touching and elbows slightly bent in an arc position directly over upper chest, contract abdominal muscles to bring your navel toward your spine. Make sure that your upper back stays in contact with the bench and the rest of your spine remains naturally curved.

➤ Keeping elbows bent to maintain a slight arc, lower arms out and downward, so that hands are at 3 o'clock and 9 o'clock, and your elbows are level with your shoulders.

➤ Keeping chest lifted throughout the movement, contract chest muscles, then bring the cable handles up and together, returning to starting position.

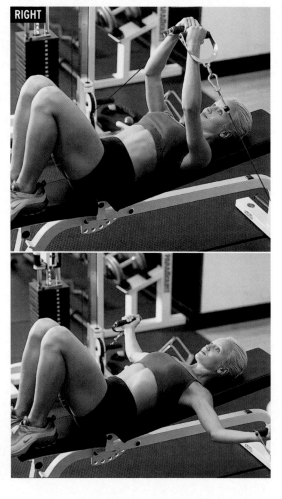

RIGHT

MUSCLES WORKED
pectoralis major, anterior deltoid

INCLINE LOW-CABLE FLY

THE PAYOFF
This move will help you develop attractive, visible definition from your collarbone to your midchest, creating a defined cleavage and more beautiful breasts. Using cables rather than dumbbells to perform this exercise also offers a more graceful, sensory experience and provides consistent resistance in both directions to work the muscles of your chest efficiently.

WORKOUT GUIDELINES
Do 2-3 sets of 8-15 reps. Rest for about 45-60 seconds between sets. Begin with 10-30 pounds on each cable, depending on the machine. Progress by increasing weight in 5-pound increments to engage and fatigue the chest, yet not recruit your arms or back to do the work.

EXPERT ADVICE
"Elevate your chest as you lift the weight," says Karen Andes, certified teacher/trainer and fitness author from Northern California. "Think of exaggerating good posture, as if you are puffing out your chest in pride like a peacock; this will help to define your cleavage."

Using cables to perform this exercise provides consistent resistance to work the muscles of your chest efficiently.

MISTAKES TO AVOID

➤ **Don't** set the incline bench at too high an angle; if you set it at more than 30 degrees when you do this move, you will be using your shoulder muscles more than your chest muscles to do the work.

➤ **Don't** lower your elbows below the level of your shoulders; this will place too much stress directly on your shoulder joint and could result in injury.

➤ **Don't** let your chest collapse at the top of the movement; remember to keep it lifted. If you let it cave in as you do the fly, your chest muscles will be doing less of the work.

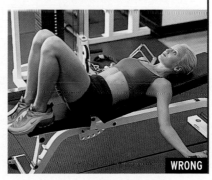

WRONG

Here's a fresh look at a classic move for building a strong upper body.

THE RIGHT WAY

➤ Kneel on floor with wrists in line with shoulders, arms straight and knees in line with hips. Extend one leg at a time behind you so you're supported on the balls of your feet and your body is in one straight line from head to heels in a "plank" position.

➤ Look straight down, neck in line with spine, fingers pointing forward and abdominals contracted, spine in a neutral position. Contract your buttocks and tighten your leg muscles along with your abs to maintain the position.

➤ Bend elbows, and lower chest toward the floor until elbows are even with shoulders, forming 90-degree angles.

➤ Press back up to the starting position, straightening, but not locking, elbows.

MUSCLES WORKED
pectoralis major, anterior deltoid, triceps

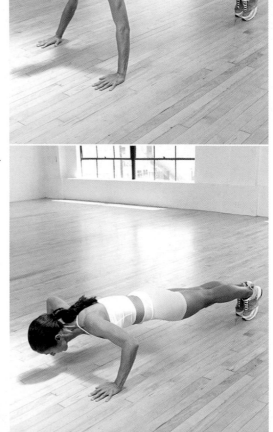

RIGHT

MILITARY PUSH-UP

THE PAYOFF

The military push-up provides more than chest-strengthening benefits. The full-body plank position requires your abdominals, hips and back to be strong enough to maintain the position as you lift and lower your body weight. You'll get more tone and visible definition in your chest and front shoulders, while adding some great shape to your triceps.

WORKOUT GUIDELINES

Start with one set of 10 reps. Do as many full push-ups as you can (up to 10) with proper form; do the rest with knees bent and on the floor, ankles crossed. To progress, add a second set of push-ups after resting 60 seconds.

EXPERT ADVICE

"Instead of trying to do 10 push-ups in a row, think about doing just one with perfect form, then two," says Susan L. Hitzmann, M.S., instructor and star of the *Crunch Boot Camp Training* video. "Before you know it, you'll be doing 10."

> The plank position requires your abdominals, hips and back to be strong enough to maintain the position.

MISTAKES TO AVOID

➤ **Don't** let your belly sag; this places excess strain on your shoulders and your spine.

➤ **Don't** collapse into your shoulder blades, which decreases the amount of upper torso strength required to perform the exercise.

➤ **Don't** lower your body so close to the ground that your arms bend more than 90 degrees. This can stress the shoulder and elbow joints, and makes it difficult to push back up to the starting position.

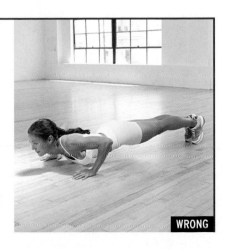

WRONG

HIP & THIGH EXERCISES

hips & thighs

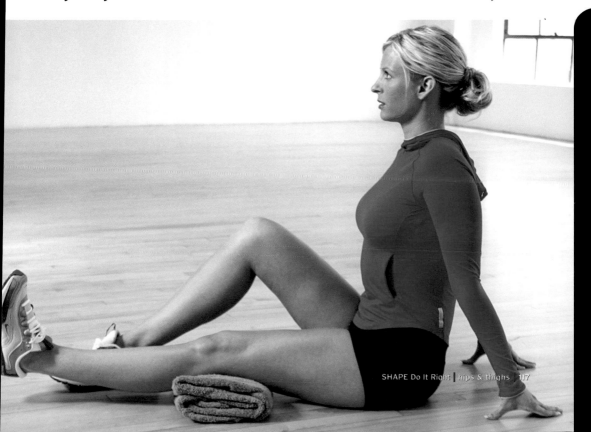

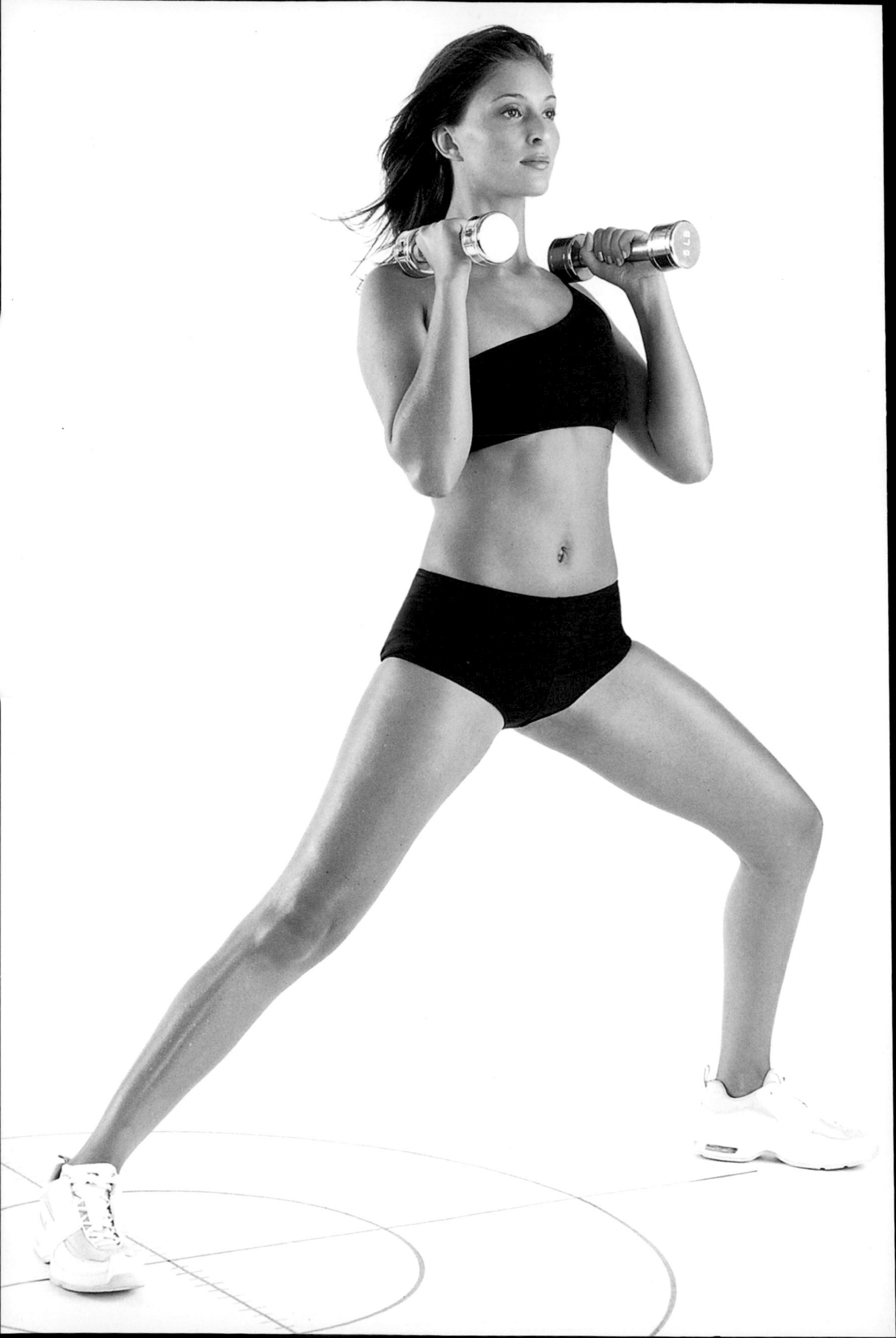

HIPS & THIGHS

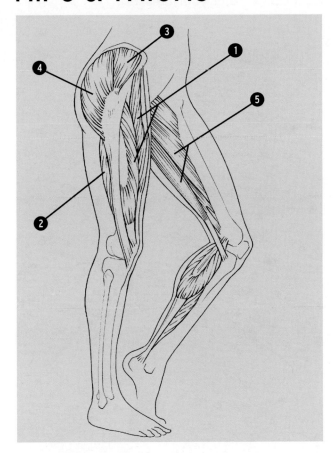

MUSCLES
1. quadriceps
2. hamstrings
3. gluteus medius
4. gluteus maximus
5. adductors

The hip and thigh muscles work with the buttocks during multi-muscle exercises. They can also be isolated and trained individually. The front thigh is comprised of four quadriceps muscles, which flex the hip and extend the knee. The rear thigh engages your three hamstring muscles, extending the hip and flexing the knee. Five adductor muscles form your inner thighs and bring your leg toward the body's midline. The iliopsoas, your hip flexors, are activated every time you bend at the hips.

The gluteal muscles forming your upper hips are called hip abductors. They attach to your pelvis and top of your thighbone and move your leg out and away from your body's midline with the help of the gluteus minimus, located underneath it. The opposite gluteus medius works to keep your pelvis from tilting when standing on one leg.

The ultimate ballet move to tone your derrière.

THE RIGHT WAY

➤ Stand with feet a bit more than hip-width apart, knees straight (not locked). Turn feet as far out as is comfortable, rotating hips outward. Tighten abs, buttocks and inner-thigh muscles. Keep spine curved naturally, knees aligned over toes and heels on the floor.

➤ Lift arms out to sides and slightly in front of you, tightening middle-back muscles. Shoulders still, rotate elbows slightly upward so they're a bit higher than wrists. Rotate wrists so palms are forward. Arms are about shoulder height.

➤ Bend knees, lowering in four counts as far as you can or until thighs are parallel to floor.

➤ Straighten legs to starting position in four counts, keeping heels on the floor.

MUSCLES WORKED
quadriceps, hamstrings, adductors, gluteus maximus

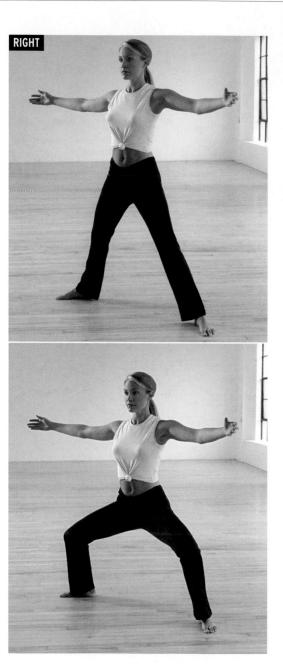

RIGHT

GRAND PLIÉ

THE PAYOFF
If you've been to the ballet, you've seen the fabulous legs of the dancers on stage. Get stronger, toned thighs, shapely hips and a dancer's derrière, with the ballerina's grand plié. Your abdominal and back muscles work hard to keep your torso centered and stable, improving your posture as well.

WORKOUT GUIDELINES
Do 2 sets of 8 pliés, resting 30 to 45 seconds between sets. To progress, either add another set or do the exercise elevated on the balls of your feet. No weight required.

EXPERT ADVICE
"Pretend you're doing pliés in a big vat of spa mud," says Rebecca Metzger, manager of the New York City Ballet Workout, who has taught at New York Sports Club and others nationwide. "Move slowly and feel the resistance against your muscles as you go up and down. Ballet is about moving in a smooth, controlled and graceful way."

Get stronger, toned thighs, shapely hips and a dancer's derrière, with the ballerina's grand plié.

MISTAKES TO AVOID
➤ **Don't** drop your hips below knee level, which can place stress on both your knees and your back.
➤ **Don't** rock hips or pelvis forward or back. This decreases the effectiveness of the exercise.
➤ **Don't** let your knees roll inward of your feet; this puts stress on the knee and knee ligaments.

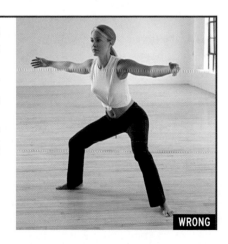

WRONG

Take a seat to strengthen your thighs without stressing your knees.

THE RIGHT WAY

➤ Roll a folded towel so that it is 6 inches in diameter. Sit on the floor with right foot flat on the floor and the towel under your left knee so that it's slightly bent, not locked. Sit erect, with fingertips on the floor behind you and pull your abdominal muscle inward and your shoulder blades together and down.

➤ Raise your left heel until the knee is straight, but not hyperextended. Keeping the leg straight, raise it slightly higher. Hold for 4 counts; lower to starting position.

➤ Concentrate on pulling the kneecap toward your hip and keeping the quadriceps tight. Keep your abs tight to avoid contracting your back.

MUSCLES WORKED
quadriceps

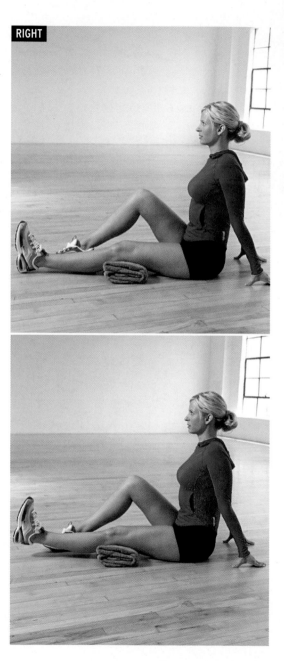

RIGHT

SEATED LEG RAISE

THE PAYOFF

A variety of factors, including weak quadriceps, make many women prone to knee problems. The seated leg raise works the quadriceps while using a limited range of knee movement. It is gentler on the knees than machine leg extensions and it requires no heavy equipment.

WORKOUT GUIDELINES

Do 8 reps, switch legs and repeat. Gradually increase to 12 reps per leg. To progress, raise the leg higher, sit in a more upright position, or add a 1- to 2-pound ankle weight, increasing a pound at a time whenever you can do 12 reps comfortably; don't exceed 8 pounds per ankle.

EXPERT ADVICE

"Concentrate on 'pulling' the kneecap toward your hip and keeping the quads tight," says Karen Clippinger, M.S.P.E., a Los Angeles-based kinesiologist and instructor at UCLA. "To feel if your muscle is contracting, place your fingertips about 2 inches inside the edge of your knee cap as you lift your leg."

The seated leg raise works the quadriceps while using a limited range of knee movement.

MISTAKES TO AVOID

➤ **Don't** lift your leg so high that your pelvis tilts under. This forces you to use your hip flexors, not your quadriceps, and it also stresses the lower back muscles.

➤ **Don't** hyperextend your knee or jam your knee straight to lift it higher; you'll put stress on the knee joint.

➤ **Don't** round your upper back or shoulders; this destabilizes your torso and gives you very little support to sit upright.

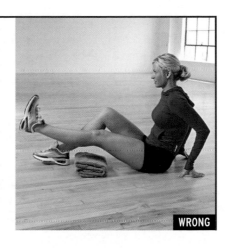

WRONG

Perfect your lunge technique for lean, toned legs and a seriously sculpted butt.

THE RIGHT WAY

➤ Stand inside a Smith machine, holding bar with an overhand grip, hands slightly more than shoulder-width apart, bar balanced on shoulders.

➤ Stagger feet about a stride's length apart, back heel lifted, abs contracted, shoulder blades pressed down and together and chest lifted.

➤ Unlock bar and lower yourself so that thigh of front leg is as parallel to the floor as possible, keeping torso erect, front knee in line with front ankle and back knee pointing down.

➤ Contract buttocks and hamstrings, pressing through front heel to straighten legs. Repeat for all reps before switching legs.

MUSCLES WORKED
quadriceps, hamstrings, buttocks, calves

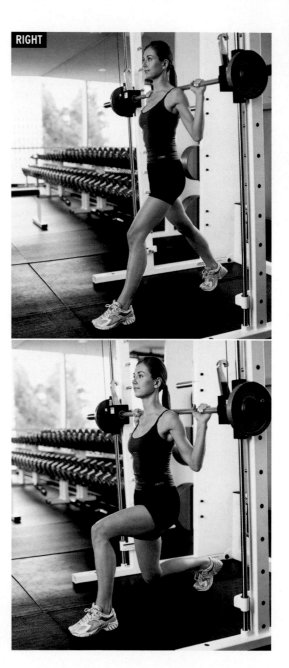

RIGHT

SMITH MACHINE LUNGE

THE PAYOFF

The alignment-perfecting assistance of the Smith machine will teach you to perform impeccable lunges without the machine. It is also a safe way to add weight to your lunges.

WORKOUT GUIDELINES

Perform 2-3 sets of 10-15 reps on each leg. Rest for 45-60 seconds after each set or continue to alternate legs, using setup time as your rest period. Use 0-25 pounds on each side, depending on machine. To progress, perform a rear lunge: Begin with both feet in front of the bar, hip-width apart, and step back about a stride's length, then bend knees, keeping rear heel lifted.

EXPERT ADVICE

"Think of this lunge as a one-legged squat, where your back leg helps stabilize the position," says Mission Viejo, Calif.-based trainer Rob Glick, B.S. , regional group fitness director for Crunch Fitness. "This will help keep your weight centered so you'll work both legs."

The assistance of the Smith machine will teach you to perform impeccable lunges without the machine.

MISTAKES TO AVOID

➤ **Don't** start with your feet too near each other; this will place stress on your knee joint, ligaments and tendons.

➤ **Don't** round your spine as you perform the lunge; this can stress the vertebrae and discs of the neck and upper back.

➤ **Don't** let your back heel make contact with the floor; this may overstretch your Achilles tendon, which can cause injury.

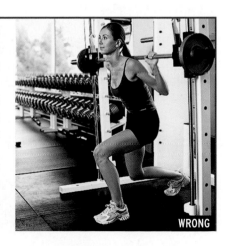
WRONG

Blast your lower body into shape with this efficient move.

THE RIGHT WAY

➤ Attach an ankle strap to your right ankle and stand on a 10-pound plate with feet together, left hip about a foot from the cable, left hand on the cable column for support and right hand on your hip.

➤ Keeping your eyes focused forward, abs tight and left knee straight, tighten your left thigh and hip muscles and lift your right toes slightly so your right ankle is in a neutral position.

➤ Initiating the move from your right hip, lift right leg out and slightly forward, making sure not to raise leg more than 30–45 degrees, while keeping knees straight but not locked.

➤ Slowly lower leg to starting position and repeat.

MUSCLES WORKED
gluteus medius

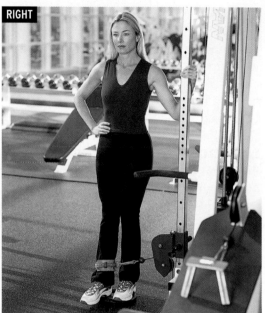

RIGHT

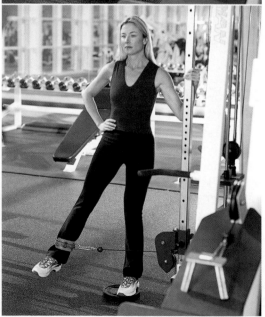

CABLE ABDUCTION

THE PAYOFF
This move works your upper hip muscles, giving your butt an extra boost. In addition to delivering a sleeker, sexier lower body, the cable abduction also stabilizes your knees, strengthens your legs and improves your balance to help you get in prime condition for cardio activities like in-line skating and kickboxing.

WORKOUT GUIDELINES
Do 2 or 3 sets of 15-20 reps on each leg. Rest 45-60 seconds between sets. To progress, alternate sets from leg to leg without rest. Suggested weight: 10-20 pounds.

EXPERT ADVICE
"As you lift up your leg, try to imagine that there's a string attached to the top of your head pulling you upward," says Mark Cibrario, owner of The Trainer's Club in Northbrook, Ill. "Staying lifted will keep you elongated in your torso and hips so you can get a greater range of motion from the lift."

The cable abduction also stabilizes your knees, strengthens your legs and improves your balance.

MISTAKES TO AVOID
➤ Don't lift your leg too high. If your standing leg starts to bend, you'll shift the work from your hips to your oblique and back muscles.
➤ Don't drop your chest or round your back. Collapsing your posture will put excess pressure on your lower back.
➤ Don't use too much weight. You'll have a tendency to lean into the weight to use other, larger muscles to do the work.

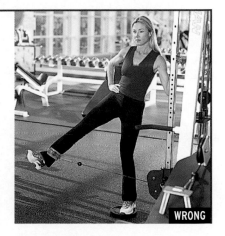
WRONG

Your inner thighs will squeeze big rewards from this easy-to-do exercise.

THE RIGHT WAY

➤ Put a 2-pound weight cuff around each ankle. Lie on your back with arms by your sides and your buttocks and the backs of your legs against the wall. Begin with your legs together and extended up toward the ceiling. Abdominal muscles are contracted.

➤ Keep your heels on the wall throughout the exercise. For about 4 seconds, move your legs apart, simultaneously lowering them toward the floor in a slow, controlled manner; you should feel a mild stretch, but no pain.

➤ Pause briefly in the bottom position. Then, slowly pull your legs back up to the starting position.

MUSCLES WORKED
adductors

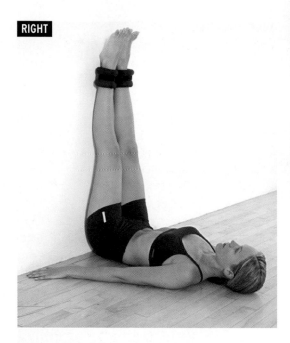

RIGHT

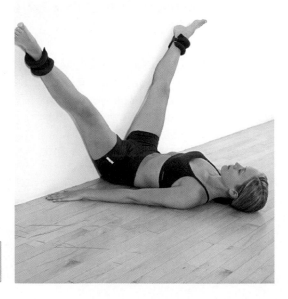

WALL ADDUCTOR

THE PAYOFF
Many women consider their inner thighs a problem zone. While excess fat may cause flabbiness, poor muscle tone also may be to blame. This move firms those hard-to-target muscles. Strong inner thighs look better than weak ones, and can prevent injuries.

WORKOUT GUIDELINES
Do 1 set of 8 reps, working up to 12 reps. When you can do 12 reps with good form, gradually increase the weights in 1- to 2-pound increments, up to 8 pounds. With each weight increase, begin with 8 reps and work up to 12.

EXPERT ADVICE
"Focus on working both legs equally by pre-contracting your inner thighs before you bring your legs together," says Karen Clippinger, M.S.P.E., a Los Angeles-based kinesiologist and instructor at UCLA. "If your hamstrings are too tight, start with your buttocks about 8 inches from the wall so your legs will be slightly bent throughout the exercise."

While excess fat may cause thigh flabbiness, poor muscle tone also may be to blame.

MISTAKES TO AVOID
➤ **Don't** rock more onto one side of your buttocks than the other; this de-stabilizes your pelvis.
➤ **Don't** arch your lower back, especially as you bring your legs together from the lower position, as this can strain your back.
➤ **Don't** separate your legs so far apart that you can't keep your legs straight or use your inner thighs to bring your legs back together.

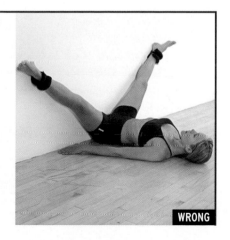

WRONG

An easy way to boost your bottom line.

THE RIGHT WAY

➤ Sit on the floor. Tie a resistance band around both legs, just above your knees. Lean back on your elbows, legs straight in front of you, ankles about 12 inches apart. Contract your abdominals and buttocks throughout the entire movement.

➤ Separate ankles about 3 feet apart, keeping legs parallel and knees pointed up.

➤ Rotate legs outward from your hips as a unit (don't let lower legs twist at knees), so knees point outward, transferring leg weight to the outside of your heels.

➤ Separate your ankles another foot apart. Hold this position for about 4 counts; then slowly return to the starting position.

MUSCLES WORKED
gluteus medius, gluteus minimus, gluteus maximus

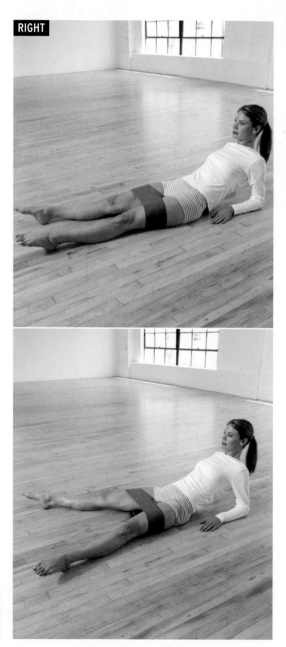

RIGHT

V HIP ROTATOR

THE PAYOFF
The V hip rotator works your buttocks and outer hips for a firm, shapely look. Leaning back on your elbows minimizes the "cheat" factor inherent in moves done standing or on your side. You'll get a tighter tush that looks great and helps you perform better in sports like hoops and running; plus, strong hip abductors stabilize your pelvis to help prevent knee and back problems.

WORKOUT GUIDELINES
Do 2 to 3 sets of 8 to 12 reps, resting 45 to 60 seconds between sets. To progress, increase your range of motion by separating legs farther apart (as long as you can maintain alignment) or switch from a medium- to a higher-resistance band.

EXPERT TIPS
"Initiate the movement from your hips, not by using your knees," says Karen Clippinger, M.S.P.E, Los Angeles-based kinesiologist and instructor at UCLA. "Make sure the band is closer to your hips than your knees; if you feel any knee pain, you're not doing the move correctly."

Leaning back on your elbows minimizes the "cheat" factor inherent in moves done standing or on your side.

MISTAKES TO AVOID

➤ **Don't** jut out your rib cage or arch your back; this places strain on the low-back muscles and connective tissue.
➤ **Don't** try to keep the kneecaps facing up rather than rolling the knees outward to follow the natural movement of your legs; this can stress your knees.
➤ **Don't** use momentum or bounce against the resistance, which can stress hip and knee joints as well as jar your back.

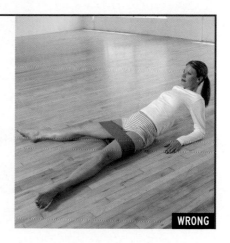

WRONG

Sculpt and define your lower body with this single-leg move.

THE RIGHT WAY

➤ Sit on a leg-press machine with the seat back adjusted to 45–60 degrees.

➤ Center one foot on plate, toes pointing straight up, in line with hip, and place other foot on floor between the seat and plate.

➤ Contract abdominals so back is in a neutral position and hips are firmly against seat, then hold handles for support, unlock machine and push plate up to straighten leg.

➤ Keeping body weight toward heel and knee aligned with second toe, bend knee in toward chest for 4 counts until it is in line with hip.

➤ Pause for 2 counts, then press through heel as you straighten leg to starting position for 4 counts; do reps, then switch legs.

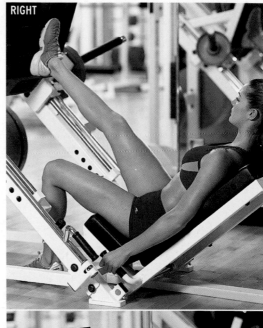

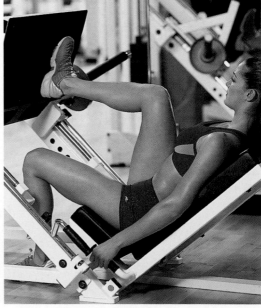

MUSCLES WORKED
quadriceps, hamstrings, gluteus maximus, adductors, gluteus medius

ONE-LEGGED PRESS

THE PAYOFF
This move ups the benefits of a leg press by working one leg at a time, causing the inner-thigh and upper-hip muscles (the adductors and abductors, respectively) to be engaged significantly throughout the movement. It also targets the quadriceps, hamstrings and gluteus maximus, so you get shapelier legs, a better butt and more balanced lower-body strength.

WORKOUT GUIDELINES
Start by adding 10-25 pounds on each side of the machine so you are lifting a total of 65-95 pounds (including the machine's 45 pounds). Perform 3-4 sets of 12 reps on both legs (1 set equals reps on both sides). To progress, as you become stronger, add 10 pounds on each side.

EXPERT ADVICE
"Gently lift your toes an inch or so away from the plate when your leg is completely extended, before beginning your next rep," says Jon Giswold, New York City-based trainer and author of *Basic Training* (St. Martin's Press, 1998). "This ensures that you're utilizing all your leg muscles with proper technique and helps target your buttocks."

This multi-muscle move ups the benefits of a leg press by working one leg at a time.

MISTAKES TO AVOID
➤ **Don't** press the plate with your toes; this can stress the knee joint.
➤ **Don't** place the seat back beyond a 60-degree angle; this position causes more spine flexion, preventing you from adequately pressing with your leg.
➤ **Don't** let the knee "wander" to either side of ankle and toes; this can change the muscles used and stress the knee joint.

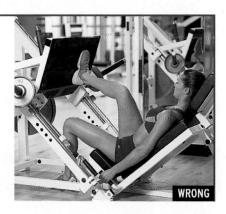

WRONG

Twist your way to tighter thighs with this ball move.

THE RIGHT WAY

➤ Put a 2- to 6-pound medicine ball just above your knees, squeeze ball to hold it in place. Stand, knees bent at about 20 degrees, abdominals contracted.

➤ Look straight ahead, and squeeze shoulder blades together. Arms are just below shoulder height, elbows bent.

➤ Keep shoulders and head facing forward, and jump up so feet leave the floor. Twist lower body to the right, landing on the balls of your feet with your feet 30–90 degrees off center. Keep knees and feet facing the same direction, without throwing your arms.

➤ Jump up and twist left. Hop right and left, like a skier doing moguls, or pivot. Squeeze the ball with inner thigh muscles.

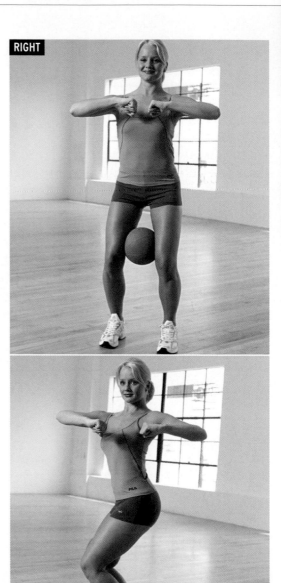

RIGHT

MUSCLES WORKED
gluteus maximus, adductors, gastrocnemius, soleus

MEDICINE-BALL TWIST

THE PAYOFF
This explosive move, which involves doing the Chubby Checker twist with a weighted ball between your legs, tones your midsection and strengthens every muscle in your lower body. It also gives you more power and agility for activities that require abrupt changes in direction, like skiing and soccer.

WORKOUT GUIDELINES
Warm up with 1 or 2 sets of 8-10 reps at moderate effort. (Twisting right, then left is one rep.) Rest 45-60 seconds between sets. Then do a set of 8-10 reps at maximum effort, jumping as high and as quickly as you can. To progress, build up to 6 all-out sets.

EXPERT ADVICE
"Your goal is to twist fast: Imagine you're jumping on a hot plate and don't want your feet to stay on the ground long so they won't get burned," says Paul Chek, a sports-conditioning specialist in Encinitas, Calif. Start with moderate effort and avoid looking down and rounding your spine, which can cause harm to your back; instead, look straight ahead.

This explosive move tones your midsection and strengthens every muscle in your lower body.

MISTAKES TO AVOID
➤ **Don't** land flat-footed, which can make your landing harder and jar your spine and other joints.
➤ **Don't** use momentum, arch your back or throw your torso side-to-side and flail your arms; this puts stress on your joints and your back.
➤ **Don't** forget to squeeze the medicine ball with your inner thighs, otherwise it will fall from the position above your knees.

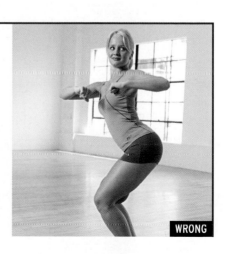

WRONG

A great move to sculpt your hips and thighs.

THE RIGHT WAY

➤ Holding dumbbells by your sides, stand with feet slightly apart, legs straight but not locked and toes pointing straight ahead.

➤ Keeping right leg straight and right toes forward, step sideways with left foot, left toes pointed at 45 degrees, bending left knee until it's in line with ankle and aligned with second toe.

➤ Keep torso centered as you lunge. You should feel a slight stretch in your inner thighs, but don't go so far that you cannot maintain an erect torso.

➤ Push back off left heel, straightening legs to starting position.

➤ Repeat for all reps; switch sides.

MUSCLES WORKED
adductors, gluteus medius, gluteus maximus, quadriceps, hamstrings

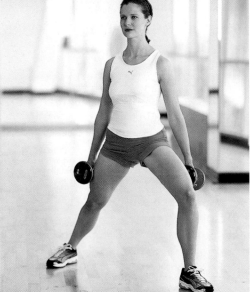

RIGHT

SIDE LUNGE

THE PAYOFF

The side lunge adds a sweep to your quadriceps and roundness to your butt. Your legs and butt will be more shapely and toned, and you'll achieve a more injury-proof, posture-perfect torso, since your back and abdominal muscles will work hard to keep you centered. What's more, you'll get more inner and outer thigh work than with a regular lunge, for both the lunging leg as well as the stabilizing leg.

WORKOUT GUIDELINES

Starting with 5- to 12-pound dumb-bells, do 2 or 3 sets of 8-15 reps, resting 45-60 seconds between sets. For a greater challenge, alternate sides on each lunge.

EXPERT ADVICE

"Make sure you use your abdominals, lift your breastbone and drop your shoulders, rather than just sidestepping into the lunge position," advises Leigh Crews, NASM, Cooper Institute-certified trainer and owner of Dynalife Fitness Inc. in Rome, Ga. "By doing so, you'll gain more control of the movement and work your leg muscles more effectively."

The side lunge adds a sweep to your quadriceps and roundness to your butt.

MISTAKES TO AVOID

➤ **Don't** angle your torso forward as you lunge; this can cause your lower back to arch and your upper back to round, stressing your lower back and causing you to lose core stability.

➤ **Don't** let your torso lean sideways into the lunge; you'll put excess pressure on the lunging knee.

➤ **Don't** let your lunging knee go past your toes or rotate inward; this can place extreme stress on the knee ligaments and tendons.

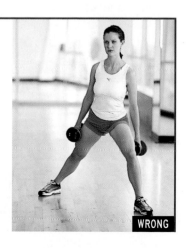

WRONG

Tone your tush with a new twist on the traditional fencing lunge.

THE RIGHT WAY

➤ Stand with heels touching, right foot pointing forward, left foot pointing sideways; hands on hips.

➤ With legs straight, step out with right foot; lead with heel, toes up. Land gently, so feet are wider than shoulder-width apart.

➤ Keeping weight balanced between feet, lunge: Bend right knee until it's in line with ankle (not over toes); keep left leg straight. Keep your back and pelvis in a neutral position, tailbone pointed toward the floor and abs tight.

➤ As you lunge, look over your right shoulder (but not behind you). In the final position, hips and shoulders are squared and open to the left (same as your left foot) with right knee and foot pointing forward.

➤ To step back, bend your left knee and push off right heel; the deeper the back-knee bend the easier it will be to recover.

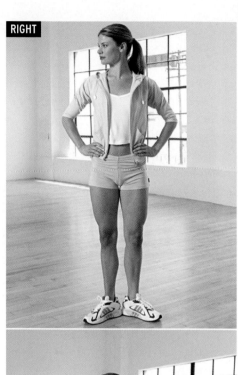

RIGHT

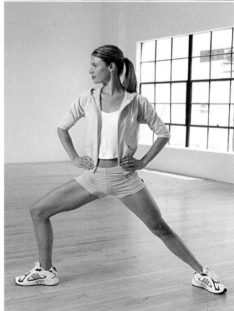

MUSCLES WORKED
quadriceps, hamstrings, gluteus medius, adductors, gastrocnemius, soleus

FENCING LUNGE

THE PAYOFF

The fencing lunge defines and strengthens all of your leg muscles and is an effective stabilization exercise. Your core muscles must work hard to keep the torso centered as you lunge. You'll get more inner thigh and upper hip work than with a regular lunge, for both the lunging leg as well as the stabilizing leg.

WORKOUT GUIDELINES

Do 1 set of 10 to 15 lunges on one leg, then switch legs and repeat. Rest 45 to 60 seconds if needed, and do another set of lunges on each leg. To progress: Lessen the back knee bend on the return phase.

EXPERT ADVICE

"This lunge should have as little impact as possible; each one should be a smooth execution, flowing laterally through the air like an arrow," says Andy Shaw, manager of the Westside Fencing Center in Los Angeles. "This visual reminds you not to slam your leg down when you land, but rather let your heel graze the ground. Fencers wear out the heels in all of their shoes."

Your core muscles must work hard to keep the torso centered as you lunge.

MISTAKES TO AVOID

➤ **Don't** rotate your hips and shoulders to face the same direction as your knee; this lessens the effectiveness of this type of lunge.
➤ **Don't** stick your butt out rather than keep your tailbone pointing downward. You'll place stress on your lower back.
➤ **Don't** bring your lunging knee past your toes which can stress the knee joint and connective tissue.

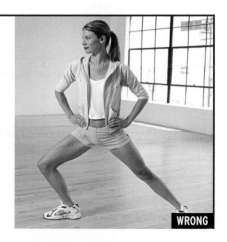

WRONG

A precision-perfect way to get killer curves and a better butt.

THE RIGHT WAY

➤ Kneeling with your right side against a stability ball, place your right elbow and forearm on the top of the ball, then lean against the ball, placing your left hand on your left hip.

➤ Keeping right knee on floor, contract abs to stabilize your torso, then extend left leg out to the side so your big toe touches the floor.

➤ Keeping your hips and shoulders square with your spine in a neutral position, lift your left leg to hip height so it's as close to parallel to the floor as possible, toes and knee pointing forward.

➤ Slowly lower your left leg to the floor, do all reps, and switch sides.

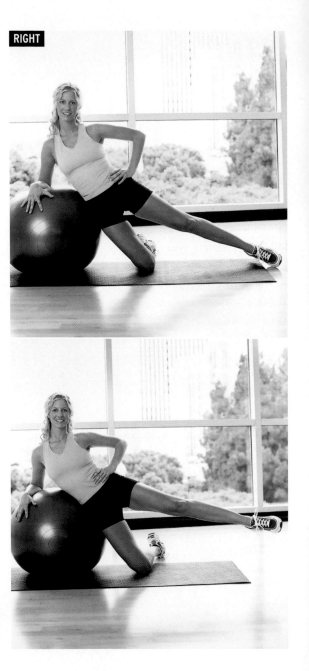

RIGHT

MUSCLES WORKED
gluteus medius, upper fibers of the gluteus maximus

SIDE-LYING BALL ABDUCTION LIFT

THE PAYOFF

Doing this move while leaning on a stability ball helps you maintain your position and comfortably lift your leg to the height necessary to isolate the appropriate muscles, so you're able to perfect your form as you strengthen and shape your hips and buttocks. Using the ball also requires torso stabilization, so as you build a shapelier lower body, your abdominals get a great workout, too.

WORKOUT GUIDELINES

Select a ball size that allows the curve of the ball to fit comfortably against your side.

Begin with 2 sets of 10-15 reps on each side, resting 1 minute between sets (after completing all reps on each side once). To progress, add a third set or use a 3- to 5-pound ankle weight.

EXPERT ADVICE

"Set your position on the ball by stabilizing with your abdominals before you lift your leg," says Lisa Wheeler, a Reebok University Master Trainer and education manager based in New York City. "This pre-set technique really helps isolate the upper hip, maximizing the toning and shaping benefits."

> The ball also requires torso stabilization, so as you build a shapelier lower body, your abdominals get a workout, too.

MISTAKES TO AVOID

➤ **Don't** use a ball that's too big for you; this will prevent you from maintaining proper balance and impede correct form.

➤ **Don't** lift your leg too high; you may lose alignment, arch your spine or lose your balance.

➤ **Don't** let your shoulders rise up to your ears or collapse your torso; this creates tension in the neck.

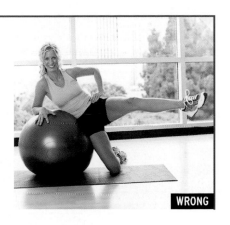

WRONG

Get ready for short skirts and outdoor sports with this thigh-tightening move.

THE RIGHT WAY

➤ Secure an ankle weight around your working ankle and hold a dumbbell in each hand, palms facing in. Stand with heels about 12 inches from a wall; rest your entire back against the wall. Keeping your left leg straight, bend your right knee so it's approximately at a 15- to 30-degree angle; raise your right thigh as high as you can toward hip height, keeping back in neutral position.

➤ Slowly bend your left knee and slide down the wall as far as you can, but not past the point at which the left thigh and knee form a 90-degree angle.

➤Hold for 5 seconds. Then, slowly straighten your left leg; sliding up the wall, return to the starting position. Do all reps, then switch sides and repeat.

MUSCLES WORKED
quadriceps, gluteus maximus, hamstrings

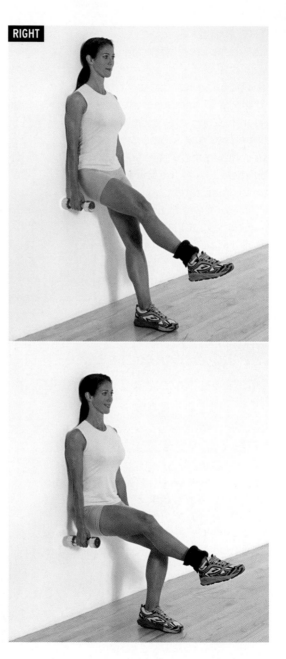

RIGHT

SINGLE-LEG WALL SLIDE

THE PAYOFF
This move strengthens and tones your thighs and butt. Because the exercise is a modified squat, it provides functional strength (meaning, it prepares you to do daily activities that involve squatting). Better yet, it works several muscles at once so it's efficient.

WORKOUT GUIDELINES
Do 2-3 sets of 8 reps on each side, working up to 12 reps each set. As you become stronger, gradually increase the depth of the squat toward 90 degrees. Begin with 5- to 10-pound dumbbells and 2- to 3-pound ankle weights. To progress, increase resistance in 1-pound increments.

EXPERT ADVICE
"Focus on keeping your abdominal muscles tight and your upper back and pelvis against the wall," says Karen Clippinger, M.S.P.E, Los Angeles-based kinesiologist and instructor at UCLA. "Avoid overarching your back as you slide up and down the wall."

Because the exercise is a modified squat, it prepares you to do daily activities that involve squatting.

MISTAKES TO AVOID

➤ **Don't** lift your leg so high that you pull your pelvis off the wall and tilt it under. This type of mistake can place undue stress on your lower back.
➤ **Don't** let the kneecap of the lifted leg roll inward, straining the knee's connective tissue.
➤ **Don't** lock your working knee when straightening your leg; this stresses the knee.

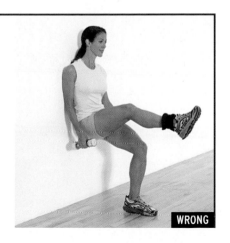

WRONG

SHOULDER EXERCISES

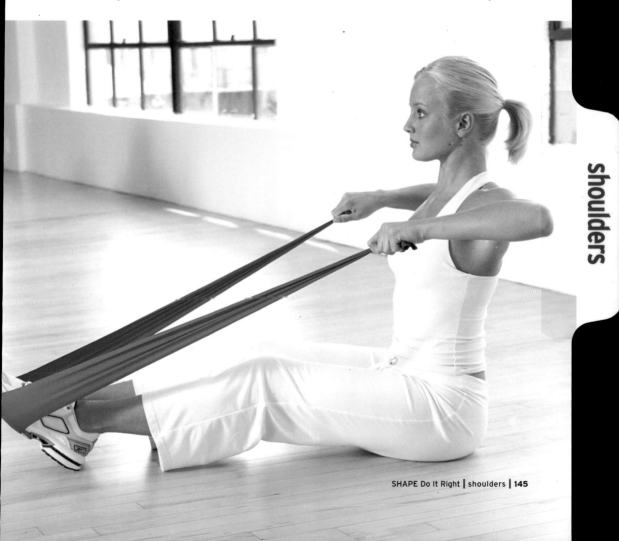

shoulders

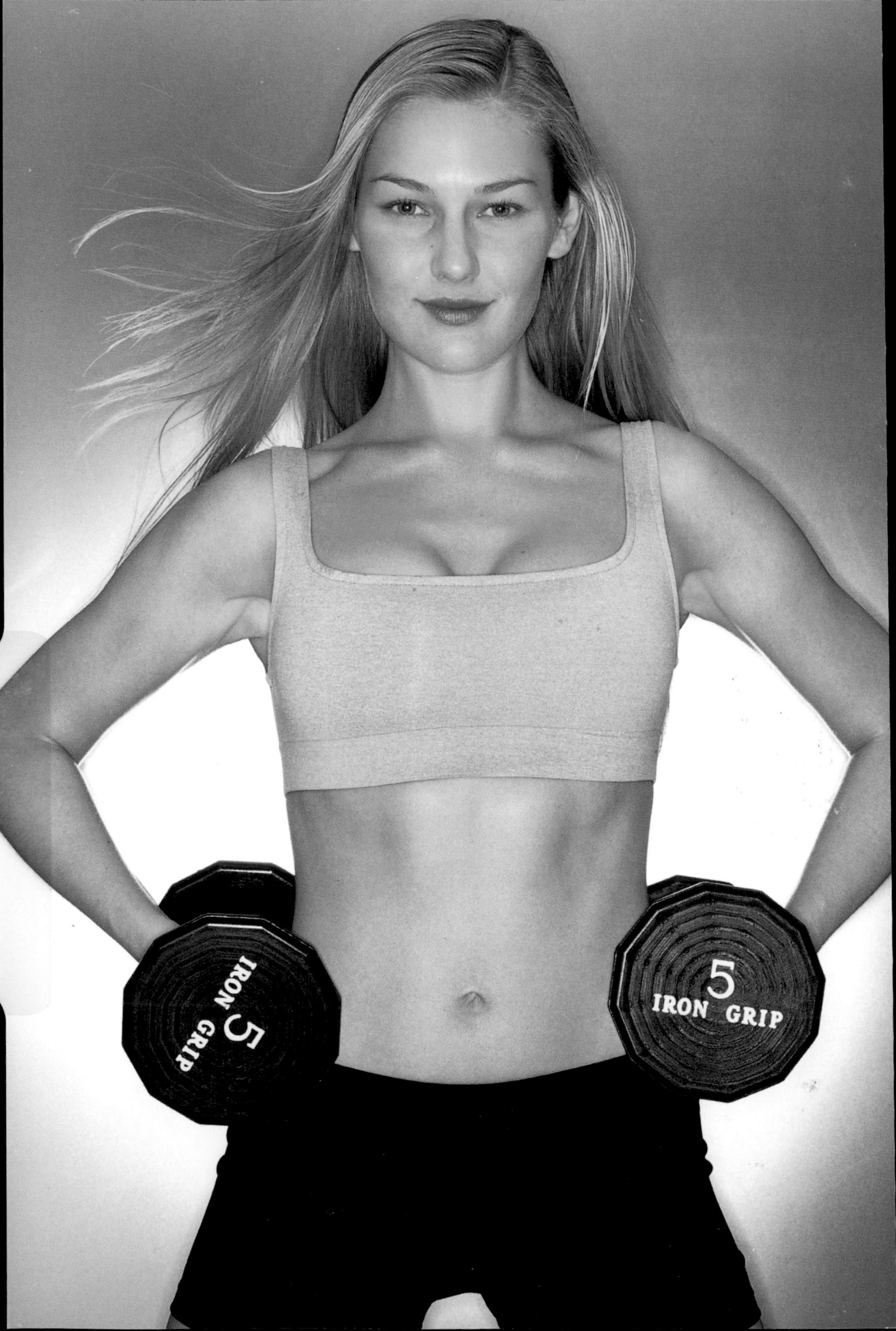
IRON 5 GRIP
5 IRON GRIP

SHOULDERS

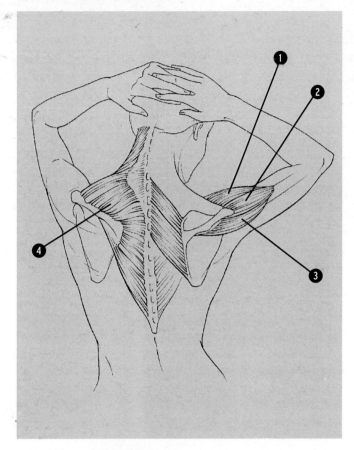

MUSCLES
1. anterior deltoid
2. lateral deltoid
3. posterior deltoid
4. trapezius

The deltoids are the triangular muscles that give shape and roundness to your shoulders. The deltoids comprise three heads that have different origins but insert at the same place on your upper arm. The anterior head at the front of your shoulder attaches on your collarbone and helps to raise your arm up and forward and rotate it inward. The posterior head is at the rear and attaches on your shoulder blade to move your arm toward the rear and rotate it outward. The lateral head, which is between the other two, lifts your arm to the side and helps the anterior and posterior heads in their movements. An accessory muscle to the deltoids that works in any overhead pressing motion is the trapezius, an upper back muscle that moves your shoulder blades.

Shrug away shoulder tension and stand a little taller with this strengthening move.

THE RIGHT WAY

➤ Sit on the edge of a bench, knees bent with feet flat on the floor, ankles in line with knees. Hold a dumbbell in each hand, arms hanging by your sides with palms facing in so wrists are aligned with shoulders.

➤ Contract your abdominals, bringing spine to a neutral position, chest lifted, shoulders down and relaxed, head aligned with neck, looking straight ahead.

➤ Without rocking your torso or changing position, slowly elevate your shoulder blades up and together, bringing your shoulders toward your ears.

➤ Pull your shoulder blades down and squeeze them together at the bottom of the movement. Lift your chest slightly to help relax the shoulder muscles between reps.

MUSCLES WORKED
trapezius

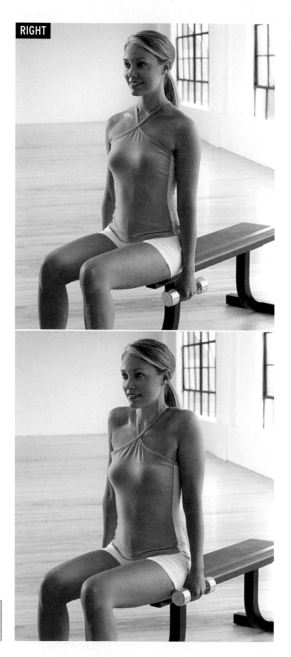

RIGHT

SHRUG

THE PAYOFF

Nagging shoulder and neck tension is a common complaint, especially among those who work at a desk. Along with everyday pressures and poor posture, you'll quickly see the wisdom of strengthening your neck and shoulders. The shrug strengthens your shoulder girdle muscles (your primary upper back stabilizers), promoting a strong postural foundation and increasing muscle endurance. It also gives you a base for developing strong, sexy shoulders.

WORKOUT GUIDELINES

Do 1 set of 8 to 10 repetitions, resting 45 to 60 seconds between sets by stretching your upper-back muscles without holding weights. To progress, add another set. Use 5- to 12-pound dumbbells in each hand.

EXPERT ADVICE

"It's more important to maintain good form than to use a heavy weight," says Debbie Ellison, Tennessee-based physical therapist and certified trainer. "If your shoulders round forward as you elevate them, use less poundage."

The shrug strengthens your shoulder girdle muscles, promoting a strong postural foundation.

MISTAKES TO AVOID

➤ **Don't** arch your lower back when shrugging. This places stress on your vertebrae and discs.
➤ **Don't** sink in your chest or allow your belly to sag; this gives you little to no torso support to perform the exercise correctly.
➤ **Don't** jut your chin out; doing so will stress your neck muscles.

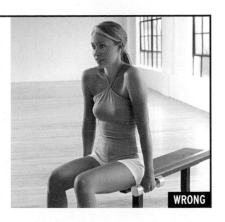

WRONG

Tone your shoulders by fine-tuning a favorite move.

shoulders

THE RIGHT WAY

➤ Hold a dumbbell in each hand with arms hanging in front of your thighs, palms facing back. Stand tall, legs straight but not locked, body weight balanced between toes and heels.

➤ Contract your abdominals to bring spine to a neutral position, chest lifted with shoulders and neck relaxed.

➤ Squeeze shoulder blades down and together to stabilize torso, then slowly raise both arms up and in front of you to shoulder height keeping wrists straight and forearms parallel.

➤ Pause at lifted position for 2 counts; then slowly lower your arms to the starting position without allowing your shoulders to roll forward.

MUSCLES WORKED
anterior deltoid

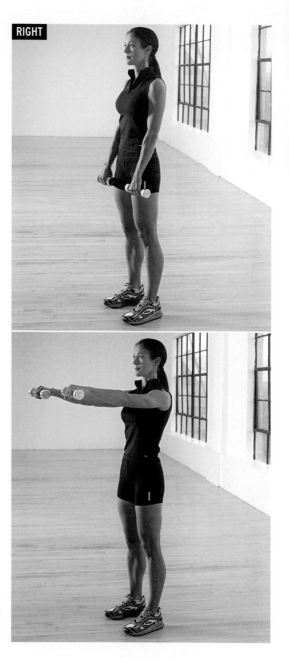

RIGHT

DUMBBELL FRONT RAISE

THE PAYOFF
Your shoulders are involved in almost every activity you do, from lifting and carrying, to most other strength-training activities and many sports. With adequate strengthening, you'll give shape to the front shoulder as well as develop more endurance to hold your arms up with less fatigue.

WORKOUT GUIDELINES
Perform 2 sets of 8 to 12 reps, resting 45 to 60 seconds between sets. When you can do 12 reps, increase your weight in 1 to 2 pound increments, decrease reps to 8 and gradually work back up to 12. Do not exceed 8 pounds in each hand.

EXPERT ADVICE
"Don't let your body weight shift back onto your heels as you lift your arms, especially if you're trying to lift with more height," says Karen Clippinger, a Los Angeles-based kinesiologist and instructor at UCLA. " Maintaining control of your torso is just as important as controlling the height of the lift."

> With adequate strengthening, you'll give shape to the front shoulder as well as develop more endurance.

MISTAKES TO AVOID

➤ **Don't** use a weight so heavy that you can't lift to at least shoulder height; this not only makes the exercise ineffective, it adds strain to upper back and shoulders.
➤ **Don't** arch or round your back as you lift; you'll stress your lower back.
➤ **Don't** drop your wrists. This places stress on the wrist and forearm muscles.

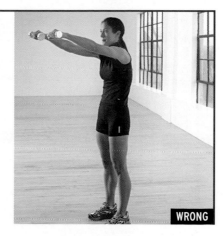

WRONG

One great move for strong, sculpted shoulders.

shoulders

THE RIGHT WAY

➤ Sit at the front of a chair with knees bent and feet flat on the floor. Hold a dumbbell in each hand, arms hanging by your sides with a slight arc to elbows, palms facing in.

➤ Contract abdominals and squeeze shoulder blades down and together to maintain neutral spine alignment in an erect sitting position. Chest is lifted and neck and shoulders are relaxed.

➤ Slowly lift arms out and up to your sides to shoulder height, no higher, without rotating arms; palms should face down at the top of the movement with wrists straight.

➤ Pause briefly at the top of the movement, then slowly lower to starting position.

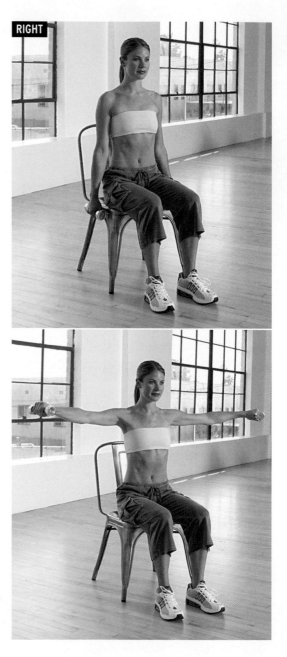

RIGHT

MUSCLES WORKED
lateral deltoid, supraspinatus

LATERAL RAISE

THE PAYOFF
This move works all the muscles of your deltoid muscle while isolating the lateral (middle), which sits on the top of your shoulder. Strong, sculpted lateral deltoids not only create a natural shoulder-pad effect, but also help with all sorts of everyday lifting and carrying motions. Any time your arms aren't hanging down by your sides, your deltoids are working, most often to aid with shoulder stability.

WORKOUT GUIDELINES
Do 2 to 3 sets of 8 to 12 reps as part of your regular strength-training program. Rest 45 to 60 seconds between sets. To progress, do the same exercise standing, which requires greater torso stabilization. Use 3- to 8-pound dumbbells in each hand.

EXPERT ADVICE
"Imagine lifting your arm out with elbows lifted rather than straight up," says Jon Giswold, New York City-based trainer and author of *Basic Training* (St. Martin's Press, 1998). "This arc-like movement ensures that your shoulders work through the full range of motion with minimal stress."

Strong lateral deltoids help with all sorts of everyday lifting and carrying motions.

MISTAKES TO AVOID

➤ **Don't** use excessive momentum to lift arms higher than shoulder height; this stresses the shoulder joint as well as delicate rotator cuff muscles.

➤ **Don't** scrunch your shoulders up to your ears as you lift. This doesn't allow you to lift through the full range of motion and also stresses your upper back and shoulders.

➤ **Don't** lock your elbows or "lift" from your wrists; you'll put undue stress on the elbow joint and forearm muscles.

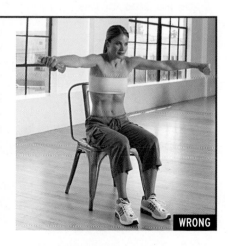

WRONG

One great move to get your shoulders strong and sculpted for sleeveless season.

THE RIGHT WAY

➤ Sit sideways on an incline bench adjusted at 45 degrees and cross one leg over the other to stack your hips and shoulders.

➤ Raise and bend your bottom arm to rest your head on it, so your neck is straight, and hold a dumbbell with your top hand, your top arm resting in line with your hip, elbow in a soft arc, palm down.

➤ Holding dumbbell, raise your arm until it is at shoulder height, no higher; pause, then lower to starting position and repeat.

➤ Before every rep, pull shoulder blades down and together, and don't let your shoulders move up toward your ears as you lift the dumbbell.

MUSCLES WORKED
lateral deltoid

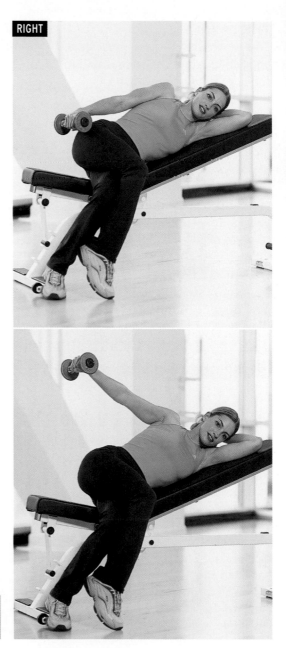

RIGHT

INCLINE SIDE-LYING LATERAL RAISE

THE PAYOFF

This move places more resistance on the shoulder muscles than typical standing exercises do so you get faster results and more definition in your middle shoulder muscle, creating a beautiful "cap" and "V" cut in the arm. You'll achieve healthy, injury-free shoulders, which are involved in virtually every upper-body exercise and activity.

WORKOUT GUIDELINES

Lift heavy one day, doing 2 sets of 8-10 reps, alternating sides, using a 6- to 8-pound dumbbell. Lift light the other day, performing 2 sets of 12-15 reps, alternating sides, using a 4- to 6-pound dumbbell. (Adjust weight to fatigue muscle by the final rep so form isn't impeded.) Progress by adding a third set.

EXPERT ADVICE

"Fix your elbow in a slightly bent position and keep it there throughout both the lifting and lowering phases," says Karen Andes, certified teacher, trainer and fitness author from Philadelphia. "This ensures that you're isolating the shoulder muscles and not using your arms or upper back to assist."

This move places more resistance on the shoulder muscles than typical standing exercises do.

MISTAKES TO AVOID

➤ **Don't** rotate dumbbells as you lift, which also engages biceps and makes the exercise less effective.
➤ **Don't** use a weight so heavy that you can't work through the full range of motion; this can stress the shoulder joint and surrounding muscles.
➤ **Don't** lift your arm too high; this impinges the shoulder joint and minimizes resistance, taking the deltoid into the "useless zone."

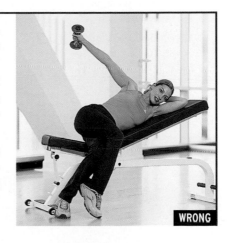

WRONG

Take a stand against weak shoulders with this strengthener.

THE RIGHT WAY

➤ Stand with your feet hip-width apart, toes either forward or slightly out, knees straight but not locked, abs tight. Hold a dumbbell in each hand at shoulder height, palms facing in, elbows pointing down. Look straight ahead and maintain body alignment from your ears down through your shoulders, hips, knees and midfoot.

➤ Take a deep breath, and then exhale as you slowly press the dumbbells upward in a slightly narrowing, triangular path, taking care to keep abs tight and torso still.

➤ Extend your arms until the weights are overhead (but not touching each other). Arms are even with ears, and elbows are straight. Pause for an instant and slowly lower the dumbbells to the starting position.

MUSCLES WORKED
anterior deltoid, lateral deltoid, trapezius

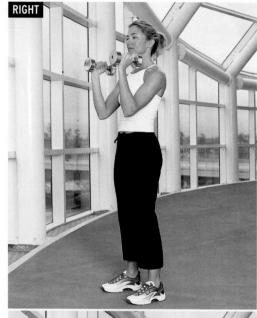

RIGHT

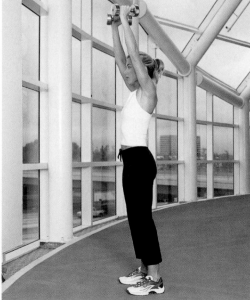

OVERHEAD DUMBBELL PRESS

THE PAYOFF

Strengthening your upper back and shoulders can make a dramatic change in your overall appearance. As you reinforce using these muscles, you'll develop a strong, confident posture and athletic looking, curved shoulders, standing taller with less fatigue and less tendency to round your shoulders because these muscles will be strong enough to support you.

WORKOUT GUIDELINES

Perform 3 to 4 sets of 8 to 12 reps, resting 45 to 60 seconds between sets. Begin with 5 to 8 pounds to perfect your overhead pressing form. To progress, increase your starting weight. Use 5 to 15 pounds.

EXPERT ADVICE

"Expect this move to be more challenging than the machine version," says trainer Juan Carlos Santana, M.Ed., C.S.C.S., owner of Optimum Performance Systems in Boca Raton, Fla. "A machine practically puts the rest of your body to sleep, but this move requires virtually all of your muscles for stabilization and balance."

Strengthening your upper back and shoulders can make a dramatic change in your overall appearance.

MISTAKES TO AVOID

➤ **Don't** lean backward and round your shoulders, a common error among those with poor shoulder flexibility. The pressure on your lower back can increase your risk of injury.
➤ **Don't** rush through the move; flinging dumbbells up and down can negate results and even cause injury.
➤ **Don't** stand with your feet too close together, limiting your stability. You need a solid base in order to press a weight that's challenging enough to strengthen and tone those delts.

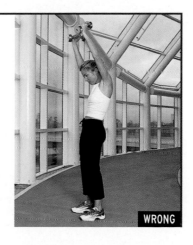

WRONG

This exercise is a sweat-free solution to slouching.

shoulders

THE RIGHT WAY

➤ Sit in a chair, elbows bent to 90 degrees and close to your sides. Grasp an elastic band with both hands. Palms face upward, wrists in neutral alignment (middle finger in a straight line with the middle of the wrist).

➤ Rotate upper arms out from shoulders so hands go away from each other. Focus on pivoting upper arms so that elbows stay by your sides while maintaining 90-degree bend (wrists in neutral alignment).

➤ Squeeze your shoulder blades together and down, then slowly lift the top of your chest toward the ceiling, so upper back arches. Concentrate on pulling the lower part of your abdomen up and back, in toward your spine, so that you avoid tilting your pelvis forward excessively.

➤ Hold for 4 counts, then slowly return to the starting position.

MUSCLES WORKED
trapezius, rhomboids, infraspinatus, teres minor, posterior deltoid, erector spinae

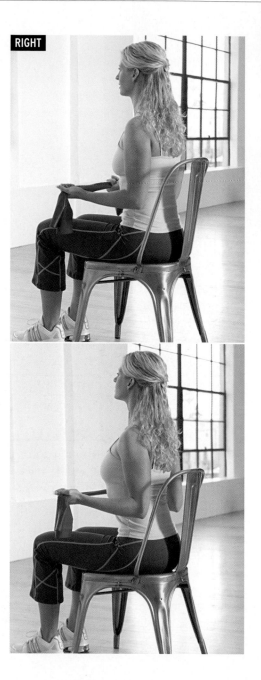

RIGHT

ROTATION ARCH

THE PAYOFF
Underdeveloped muscles in your upper back region can cause your shoulders to roll forward. The rotation arch can help strengthen your upper back and posterior shoulder muscles using a resistance band. This simple move can balance out chest and anterior shoulder muscles or, after long periods of sitting, help relieve discomfort.

WORKOUT GUIDELINES
Repeat the entire sequence 6 times, working up to 12 repetitions. When you can do 12 reps with correct form and full range of motion, gradually increase the resistance by taking a narrower grip on the band without decreasing the range of the arms. Each time you increase resistance, begin with 6 reps working back up to 12.

EXPERT ADVICE
"Focus on pivoting your upper arms so that your elbows stay in place by your sides," says Karen Clippinger, M.S.P.E., a Los Angeles-based kinesiologist and instructor at UCLA. "This way, you should feel the muscular contraction centered in your mid-and upper back, not your lower back."

This move can balance out chest and anterior shoulder muscles or, after long periods of sitting, relieve discomfort.

MISTAKES TO AVOID
➤ **Don't** arch your lower back as you pull your arms open; this places stress on your lower back muscles and spine.
➤ **Don't** move your upper arms or your elbows away from your sides. This makes the exercise an arm strengthener rather than a back strengthener.
➤ **Don't** lean your back so far that you lose the engagement of your abdominals and allow your pelvis to tilt forward excessively.

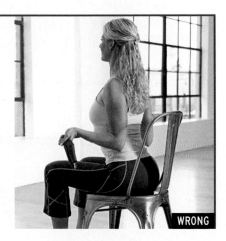

WRONG

This is the move to do when your front is stronger than your back.

THE RIGHT WAY

➤ Sit on the floor with your legs outstretched, knees slightly bent and heels on the floor.

➤ Wrap a resistance band around both feet, holding one end in each hand, palms down. Keeping your back as erect as possible, bend knees farther.

➤ Take 4 seconds to pull your elbows back until they are at shoulder height and bent to form right angles. Concentrate on pulling your shoulder blades slightly down and firmly together. Hold this position for 4 seconds then return to the starting position.

➤ Throughout the exercise, keep your shoulders over your hips while contracting your abdominal muscles to avoid overarching your back.

MUSCLES WORKED
trapezius, teres minor, infraspinatus, latissimus dorsi, lateral deltoid, posterior deltoid, teres major and rhomboids

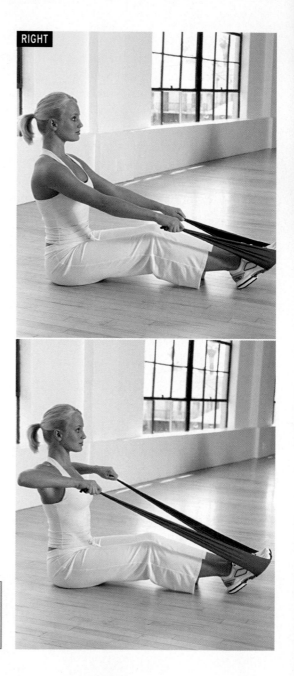

RIGHT

SEATED ROW

THE PAYOFF
Unless you specifically target the rear shoulder muscles in your workouts, you may suffer the consequences of imbalance: rolled-shoulder posture and upper-back aches. This modified seated row is a simple move that fights this imbalance by strengthening and defining your upper back and rear shoulders.

WORKOUT GUIDELINES
Start with 8 reps, and work up to 12. When you can do 12 with correct form, gradually increase the resistance by choking up on the band. Ultimately, you can graduate to using a band with more resistance or to using two bands at once. Each time you add resistance, begin with 8 reps, and work up to 12. Progress by adding a second set.

EXPERT ADVICE
"Keep shoulders over hips while contracting abdominal muscles to avoid overarching your back," says Karen Clippinger, M.S.P.E, a Los Angeles-based kinesiologist and instructor at UCLA. "If you're leaning back, you're using body weight to pull the band and not challenging your rear shoulders as effectively as you could be."

This seated row is a move that fights imbalance by strengthening and defining your upper back and shoulders.

MISTAKES TO AVOID
➤ **Don't** lift your hands too high and drop your elbows; you'll strain your forearm muscles and shoulder joints.
➤ **Don't** rock your torso; this causes stress on your back.
➤ **Don't** tuck your tailbone under. This position will compromise your posture, making it difficult to sit erect.

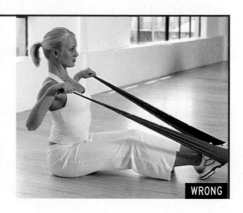

WRONG

Round out your shoulder training with this balancing act.

THE RIGHT WAY

➤ Sit on the edge of a chair, knees bent and feet flat on floor with legs separated hip-width apart.

➤ Hold a dumbbell in each hand with elbows bent at right angles, even with shoulders, forearms parallel and knuckles pointing down toward the floor. Squeeze shoulder blades together and tightly contract abdominals to maintain upright position.

➤ Without changing arm position, rotate arms from the shoulders to raise hands to chest height, then continue to rotate arms upward until knuckles point up at the ceiling.

➤ Hold for four counts then lower to start position.

MUSCLES WORKED
posterior deltoid, trapezius, rhomboids, supraspinatus, infraspinatus, teres minor

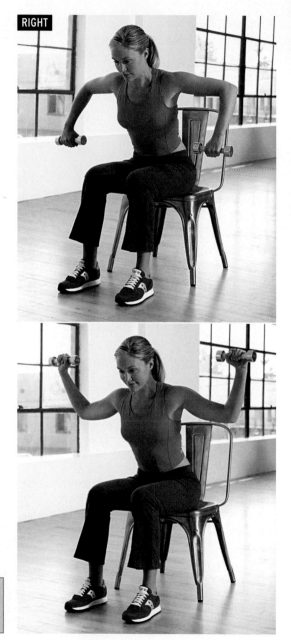

RIGHT

ROTATION FLY

THE PAYOFF
The back of the shoulder is an easy area to overlook in your strength-training routine. The rotation fly strengthens the posterior head of the deltoid (rear shoulder) as well as the rotator cuff muscles of the shoulder and the scapular adductors of the upper back. This exercise is particularly valuable for people who spend long hours working at a computer or who do a lot of lifting or sports that involve overhead arm work.

WORKOUT GUIDELINES
Do 2 sets of 10 to 12 reps, working up to 12 as part of your regular strengthening program. Rest 45 to 60 seconds between sets. To progress, increase weight in 1-pound increments. Use 3 to 8 pound weights.

EXPERT ADVICE
"For best results, go slowly and keep your spine lengthened says Karen Clippinger, M.S.P.E, a Los Angeles-based kinesiologist and instructor at U.C.L.A "Create as much space as possible between your shoulders and your ears by keeping your shoulders pressed down."

This exercise is particularly valuable for people who spend long hours working at a computer.

MISTAKES TO AVOID

➤ **Don't** drop your elbows as you rotate your upper arms; this takes the work away from the rotator cuff and shoulders, placing it instead on your back.

➤ **Don't** use momentum when lifting your arms; you can strain delicate shoulder tissue as well as the shoulder joint.

➤ **Don't** arch your back, which causes tension and strain in your lower back.

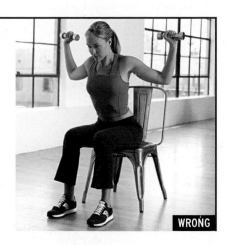

WRONG

STRETCHING EXERCISES

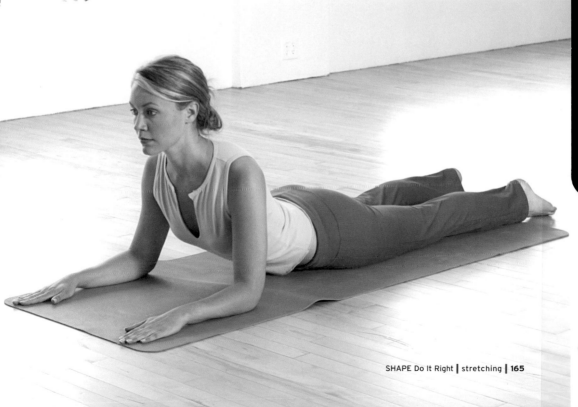

stretching

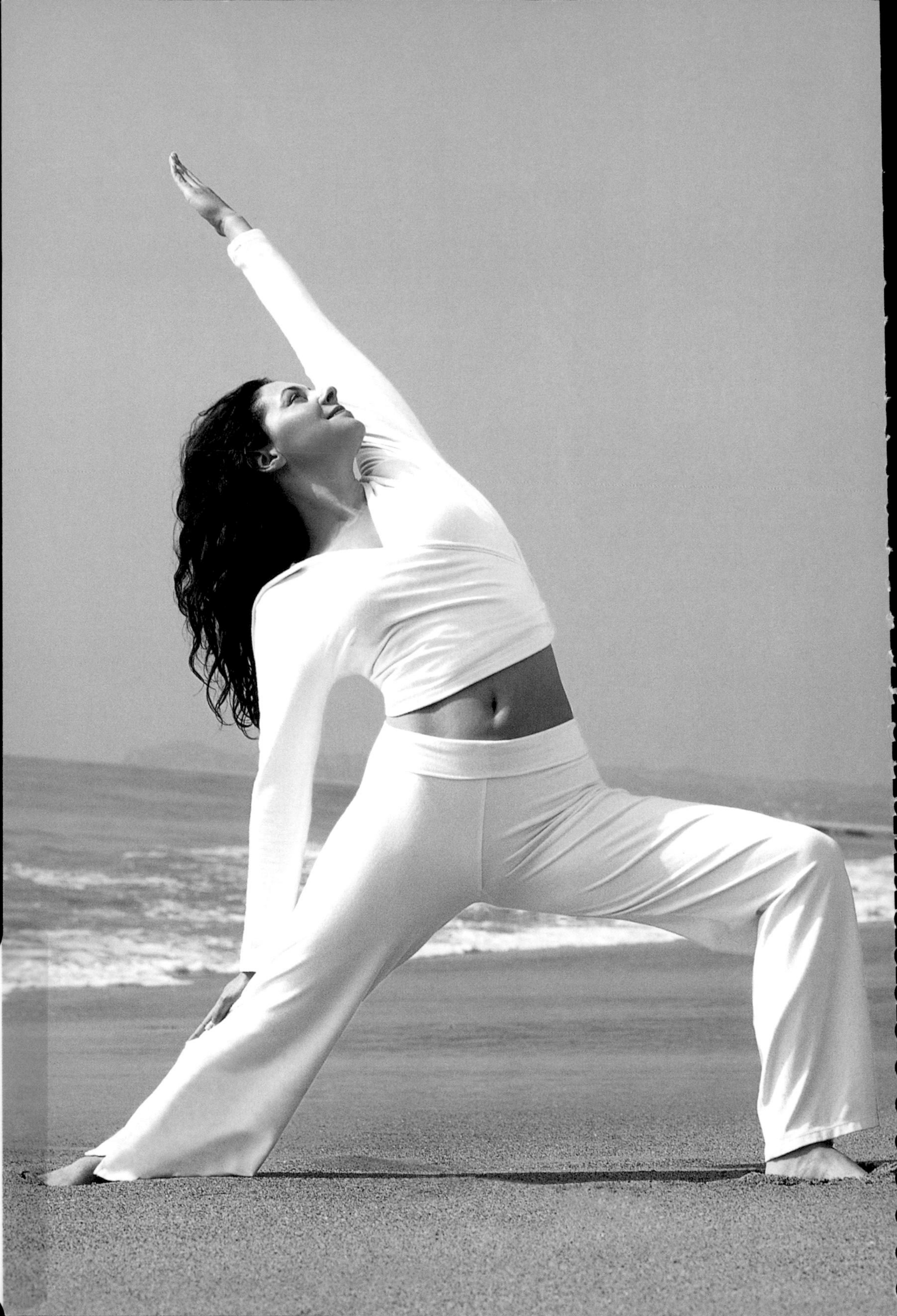

STRETCHING

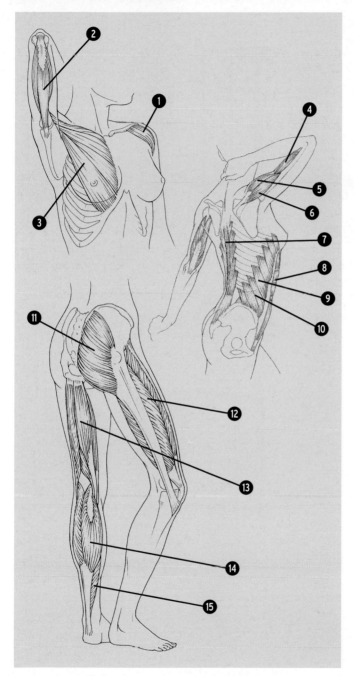

MUSCLES
1. anterior deltoid
2. triceps
3. pectoralis major
4. biceps
5. lateral deltoid
6. posterior deltoid
7. erector spinae
8. rectus abdominus
9. external obliques
10. internal obliques
11. gluteus maximus
12. quadriceps
13. hamstrings
14. gastrocnemius
15. soleus

A single, simple lunge to relax your calves and hips.

stretching

THE RIGHT WAY

➤ Stand in a lunge position with your left foot back and your hands on a wall or post for balance. Keep your right knee slightly bent and left knee straight but not locked. Your toes should point straight ahead.

➤ Slowly shift your body weight forward, letting your right knee bend a little more until you feel a stretch in your left calf and the front of your left hip.

➤ Focus on keeping your abdominal muscles tight and pressing the bottom (not the top) of the pelvis forward so your lower back doesn't arch. Think about pressing your left heel down and back to fully extend (but not hyperextend) your knee.

MUSCLES STRETCHED
gastrocnemius, iliopsoas

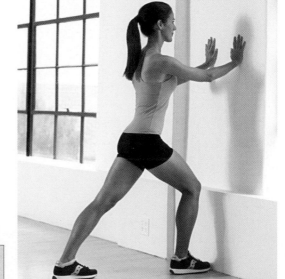

RIGHT

LUNGE FOR CALVES

THE PAYOFF

Inadequate or uneven calf flexibility could lead you to compensate by rolling your feet inward excessively, which can contribute to injuries such as shinsplints and Achilles' tendinitis. The classic lunge stretch is an effective way to improve calf flexibility. By doing it with your torso upright, you'll also get a good stretch in the hip-flexor muscles.

WORKOUT GUIDELINES

Hold the stretch for 20 to 30 seconds, concentrating on relaxing and lengthening the calf and hip-flexor muscles. Repeat two to three times on each leg, alternating sides. As hip flexors and calves become more flexible, increase the stance of your lunge if possible, as long as you can keep your heel down and hips pressed forward.

EXPERT ADVICE

"Keep your abdominal muscles tight and press the bottom, not the top, of the pelvis forward," says Karen Clippinger, M.S.P.E., a Los Angeles-based kinesiologist and instructor at UCLA. "This will prevent your lower back from arching and increase the stretch to the front of your hip."

Because the calf muscles absorb forces during many activities, it's important to keep them well-stretched.

MISTAKES TO AVOID

➤ **Don't** lunge so deeply that your front knee moves past your toes; this can stress the knee joint as well as the knee ligaments and tendons.

➤ **Don't** arch your back, putting stress on the lower spine. This also inhibits stretching your hip flexors along with your calves.

➤ **Don't** raise your back heel up off the floor, which can prevent an adequate stretch of your calves.

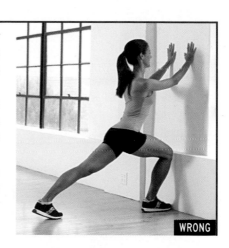

WRONG

An easy-balance stretch to relieve muscle soreness and prevent injury.

THE RIGHT WAY

➤ Sit sideways on a chair so your right side faces the back of it. Your right knee is bent about 90 degrees, and your right foot is flat on the floor. Your left leg should hang over the side. Bend your left knee (so heel moves toward your buttocks) and grasp your left foot with your left hand.

➤ Firmly contract your abdominal muscles so that your torso is stable and your pelvis is in a neutral position; slowly move your knee backward until your left knee points down toward the floor.

➤ Then, use your left hand to bring your left heel toward your buttocks until you feel a moderate stretch, but no pain, along the front of your thigh.

MUSCLES STRETCHED
quadriceps

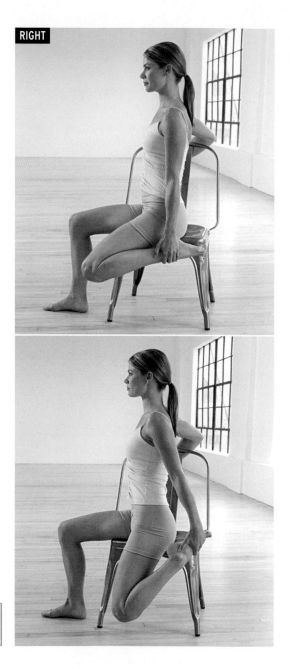

RIGHT

QUAD STRETCH

THE PAYOFF

Giving your quads a good stretch after your workout can help relieve soreness and prevent tightness. Unlike other quad stretches, this move doesn't require you to stay balanced on one foot; instead, sit on a chair.

WORKOUT GUIDELINES

Hold the stretch for 20-30 seconds as you concentrate on relaxing your thigh and pulling your knee back and down toward the floor. Perform the stretch 2-3 times on your left; repeat on the right side. To progress, as you become more flexible, aim to increase the stretch so your knee points directly toward the floor in line with your shoulder and hip.

EXPERT ADVICE

"Contracting your buttocks and hamstrings first will help you move your leg into the stretching position easier," says New York City-based Reebok University Master trainer Lisa Wheeler. "When opposition muscles contract, it makes it easier for the muscles you're trying to stretch (in this case the quadriceps) to relax."

Giving your quads a good stretch after your workout can help relieve soreness and prevent tightness.

MISTAKES TO AVOID

➤ **Don't** twist your lower leg or foot in an attempt to get a deeper stretch. This only adds torque to your ankle joint and stress to the ligaments.
➤ **Don't** arch your back or try to pull your leg up too high toward your buttocks, placing stress on both your lower back as well as the knee joint.
➤ **Don't** tilt your pelvis under, causing your shoulders to round. You'll destabilize your back, which makes it difficult to contract the abdominals.

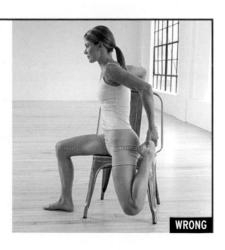

WRONG

Here's a convenient stretch that will give your legs a greater range of motion.

THE RIGHT WAY

➤ Stand erect with right heel on a chair or bench, low enough to allow you to bend forward comfortably and keep the right leg straight, toes pointed.

➤ Keeping both legs straight without locking your knees, contract abdominals and hinge forward from hips, lowering chest toward the center of right thigh until you can place your hands on either side of right foot with back straight, head and neck aligned with your spine and hips square.

➤ If keeping your leg or back straight is difficult, place your hands on your lower leg so you can maintain alignment.

➤ Hold stretch for recommended seconds, then switch legs and repeat with other leg.

MUSCLES STRETCHED
hamstrings

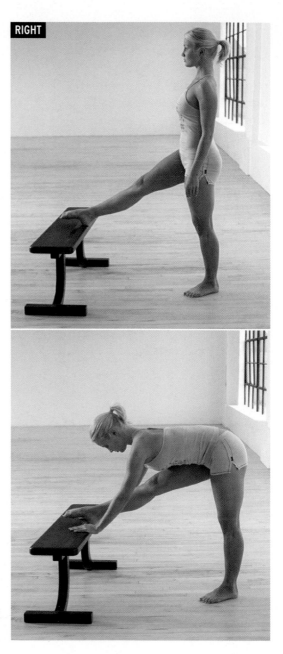

RIGHT

STANDING HAMSTRING STRETCH

THE PAYOFF

The standing hamstring stretch, more convenient and less awkward than the seated version, helps to isolate and stretch hamstrings effectively. When your hamstrings are sufficiently stretched, lower-body training will be improved, plus you'll have a better range of motion for activities such as running, dancing, stairclimbing, elliptical training and yoga.

WORKOUT GUIDELINES

Hold the stretch at a point of mild tension for 30 to 60 seconds, without bouncing, on each leg. Slowly inhale and exhale, using the exhale portion to move deeper into the stretch. Stretch each leg 2 or 3 times. To progress, walk your hands farther forward on the chair or bench to deepen the stretch.

EXPERT ADVICE

"To lengthen your spine, think of drawing your tailbone out behind you without arching your back," says Karen Clippinger, M.S.P.E., a Los Angeles-based kinesiologist and instructor at UCLA. "This will prevent your back from rounding and give you a fuller range of motion to stretch your hamstrings."

When your hamstrings are sufficiently stretched, lower-body training will be improved.

MISTAKES TO AVOID

➤ **Don't** drop your head or hunch your shoulders up toward your ears; you'll stress both the neck and back muscles, and also inhibit keeping the leg to be stretched straight.

➤ **Don't** hyperextend your knee in order to stretch farther or to keep it straight; this places undue pressure on the knee joint and its attachments.

➤ **Don't** use a support that is so high, it makes it difficult for you to keep your hips and shoulders square.

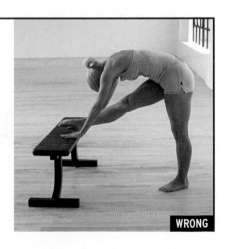

WRONG

Stiff back? Here's the soothing stretch that will provide relief.

THE RIGHT WAY

➤ Lie on your back with your right arm outstretched to your side at shoulder height, left knee bent and left foot on the floor, about 18 inches from your buttocks.

➤ Bring your right knee up toward chest and place your left fingers on the outside of your right thigh, close to the knee.

➤ Keeping upper back stationary and shoulder blades on the floor, use your left hand to pull your right knee slowly across your body and toward the floor, too. Legs and hips should twist as a unit until your weight is on the outside of your left hip. You should feel a stretch along your back and outer right hip.

➤ Hold and repeat on opposite side.

MUSCLES STRETCHED
erector spinae, gluteus medius

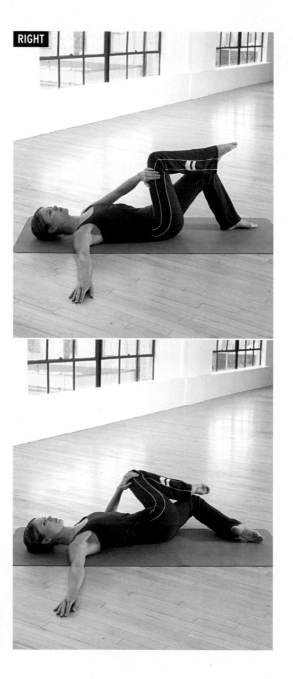

RIGHT

SPINAL TWIST

THE PAYOFF

Whether you sit behind a desk all day, spend hours in your car or repeatedly bend over to do household chores, you may experience a stiff, tired back that cries for relief. To the rescue is the spinal twist. It makes your back feel better, improves your flexibility and enhances spinal rotation by stretching the muscles through the length of the spine. Maintaining good spinal rotation can help prevent back pain and injuries.

WORKOUT GUIDELINES

Hold the stretch for 20-30 seconds, relaxing your buttocks and upper hip. Repeat 2-3 times on each side. To progress, try to move deeper into the stretch by bringing your knee closer to the floor.

EXPERT ADVICE

"To really get the most out of this stretch, focus on technique and stretch slowly without jerking," says Karen Clippinger, M.S.P.E., a Los Angeles-based kinesiologist and instructor at UCLA. "By using your hand to bring your knee across your body, you'll also stretch the muscles of your buttocks and hip."

Maintaining good spinal rotation can help prevent back pain and injuries.

MISTAKES TO AVOID

➤ **Don't** pull on your knee, dropping it so low toward the floor that it strains your lower back; if you feel pain you've stretched too far.

➤ **Don't** roll over onto your side, lifting your shoulders off the floor. This will cause tension in your neck, shoulders and upper back.

➤ **Don't** arch your back and allow your abdomen to protrude; you'll have little to no spine support as you move into the twist.

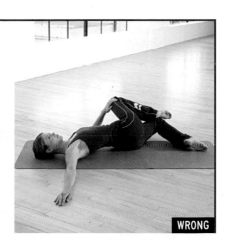

WRONG

Loosen up to help thwart back soreness with one easy move.

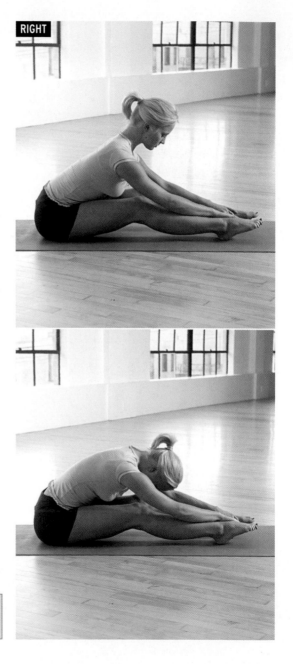

RIGHT

stretching

THE RIGHT WAY

➤ Sit on the floor or a mat with your legs stretched out in front of you, ankles six inches apart and knees slightly bent. Resting your forearms on your shins, grasp the insides of your feet.

➤ Exhale and slowly bend your elbows, using your arms to pull your spine forward and down gently. Tuck your head in, and round your back until you feel a mild to moderate stretch in your lower back.

➤ Throughout the stretch, concentrate on firmly pulling your abdominal wall inward. Also, keep your lower back as rounded as possible by bringing your head down toward the floor.

MUSCLES STRETCHED
erector spinae

FORWARD SPINAL BEND

THE PAYOFF
The muscles that support your lower back are called into action in almost everything you do. Standing in one place or sitting for long periods can put you at a greater risk for lower-back pain. The forward spinal bend can help relieve achy low-back muscles and prevent them from becoming tight in the first place.

WORKOUT GUIDELINES
Hold the stretch for 20–30 seconds, slowly breathing in and out. Concentrate on relaxing your lower back while bringing your head slightly closer to the floor with each exhale. Return to the starting position briefly, then repeat the stretch 2 more times. As your lower back becomes more flexible, increase the stretch by bringing your head closer to your knees while keeping lower back rounded.

EXPERT ADVICE
"If you aren't flexible enough to perform the exercise comfortably, place a towel around your feet and grasp the end of it," says Karen Clippinger, M.S.P.E., a Los Angeles-based kinesiologist and instructor at UCLA. "This allows you to gradually increase the forward bend."

The forward spinal bend can help relieve achy low-back muscles and prevent them from becoming tight.

MISTAKES TO AVOID
➤ **Don't** let your belly sag which inhibits using your abdominal muscles to protect your back.
➤ **Don't** straighten your back as you reach forward. This pulls on your lower back muscles and places excess strain on your vertebrae and discs.
➤ **Don't** forget to bend your knees; if you have tight hamstrings as well as inflexible back muscles, this stretch will be difficult to perform with straight legs.

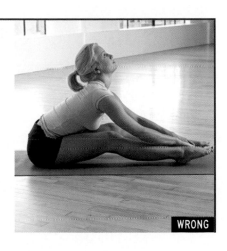

WRONG

For a healthier, supple spine, try a new take on a yoga classic.

THE RIGHT WAY

➤ Lie facedown on a mat with your arms stretched overhead. Pressing against the floor with your forearms, lift your head off the floor and walk your elbows back a few inches at a time until they're directly below your shoulders. Don't let your hips lose contact with the floor.

➤ Pull your shoulder blades down and slightly together. Focus on keeping your hips on the floor, relaxing your back muscles and letting your arms support your spine. Let your lower back sink toward the floor, and keep your head in line with your spine.

➤ Hold for 20-30 seconds, then lower your head and torso to the floor without moving your hands.

MUSCLES STRETCHED
rectus abdominis

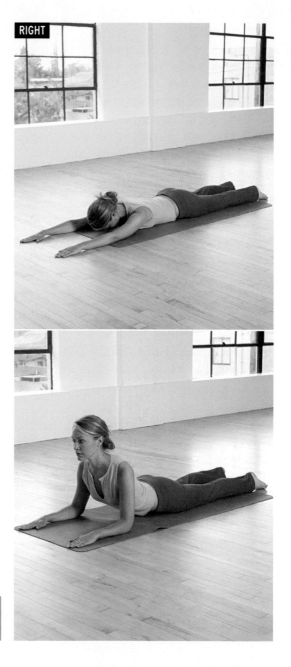

RIGHT

SPHINX

THE PAYOFF

Cultivating spinal strength and flexibility may be an important way to prevent low-back injury, as long as you do it safely. This modified version of the classic cobra provides a gentle and easy-to-control torso stretch. To round out your training program, try this stretch between abdominal exercises or as part of your regular stretching routine. This stretch can also improve the overall suppleness of your entire spine.

WORKOUT GUIDELINES

Hold the stretch for 20 to 30 seconds. Repeat 2 to 3 times. To progress, do this same exercise by straightening elbows into a true cobra position.

EXPERT ADVICE

"Keep your hips on the floor so that your back muscles fully relax," says Karen Clippinger, M.S.P.E., a Los Angeles-based kinesiologist and instructor at UCLA. "By letting your arms support your spine, you'll alleviate tension from your lower back and can achieve a more effective stretch for the front of your torso."

This modified version of the classic cobra provides provides a gentle and easy-to-control torso stretch.

MISTAKES TO AVOID

➤ **Don't** arch your back too high or press up too forcefully, causing stress to the back muscles and connective tissue as well as the vertebrae and discs.

➤ **Don't** lift your hips up off the floor rather than allowing the lower back to curve; this places additional stress on the spine.

➤ **Don't** hyperextend your neck, placing strain on the cervical spine as well as the upper back and neck muscles.

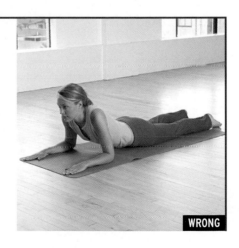

WRONG

Relieve neck tension with this simple stretch.

THE RIGHT WAY

➤ Sitting on a bench, take hold under the bench with your right hand and pull up on it gently. To ensure that your right shoulder stays down, keep your right elbow slightly bent and shoulder blade pulled downward. Maintain a firm grasp under the bench so that your shoulder blade is held stationary throughout the stretch.

➤ Place your left hand on the right side of your head. Keeping chin close to chest, slowly pull head slightly forward and to the side so that left ear moves down toward the front of left shoulder.

➤ Continue until you feel a mild stretch in the back of the right side of your neck.

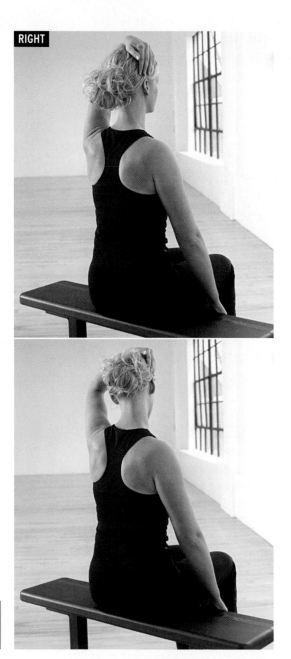

RIGHT

MUSCLES STRETCHED
lateral neck flexors, trapezius, levator scapulae

NECK STRETCH

THE PAYOFF

In addition to the role neck muscles play in times of tension, the muscles in the side and back of the neck are constantly being utilized to move and turn your head. Because these muscles also attach to the shoulder blades, they support the shoulders and assist with lifting the arms. This stretch can help relieve tightness and prevent discomfort from becoming a chronic pain in the neck.

WORKOUT GUIDELINES

Hold the stretch for 20 to 30 seconds, relaxing and allowing the neck muscles to lengthen. Switch sides and repeat. Do this move 2 to 3 times per side.

EXPERT ADVICE

"By holding onto the chair or bench with the opposite hand, you provide a gentle resistance to stretch against," says Karen Clippinger, M.S.P.E., a Los Angeles-based kinesiologist and instructor at UCLA. "This will allow you to gently keep your shoulder pulled down and away from your ear so you get a deeper stretch to your neck."

This stretch can help relieve tightness and prevent discomfort from becoming a chronic pain in the neck.

MISTAKES TO AVOID

➤ **Don't** pull on your head too hard or too fast; this strains the neck and upper spine.

➤ **Don't** jut your chin out and forward, throwing your upper spine out of alignment and decreasing the effectiveness of the stretch.

➤ **Don't** round or hunch your shoulders or slouch your torso so you can't get any range of motion to the stretch for your neck.

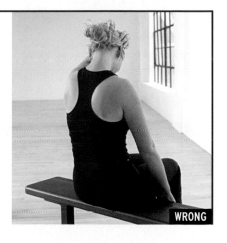

WRONG

Improve your posture with this innovative stretch.

THE RIGHT WAY

➤ Sit on an exercise ball, knees bent, feet on the ground, arms by your sides. (Or lie faceup with the top of your head at the top edge of a horizontal bench.)

➤ Curl your torso backward, contracting your abdominals to control the lowering. Keep abdominals tight throughout the move to prevent your lower back from arching.

➤ Reach arms overhead, palms up. Relax shoulders; let your arms' weight bring your hands close to the ground. Keep elbows slightly bent.

➤ Use your feet to adjust your position so that your hands almost touch the ground and your head is supported by the ball. You should feel a moderate stretch.

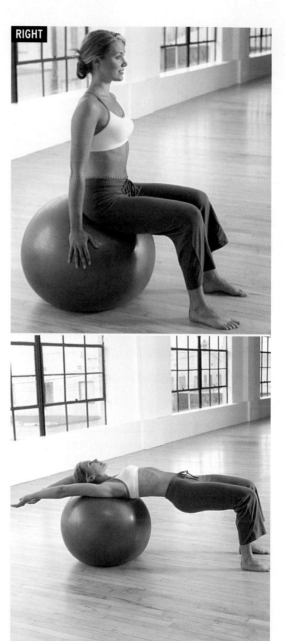

RIGHT

MUSCLES STRETCHED
latissimus dorsi, pectoralis major, anterior deltoid

SHOULDER AND CHEST REACH

THE PAYOFF

This reach can stretch your shoulder muscles even more thoroughly than a traditional shoulder stretch done seated or on the floor. The move is especially effective if you're flexible; it lets your arms stretch farther than usual while supporting your back and neck. Because tight shoulder muscles can cause your shoulders to hunch forward, increased flexibility will help "open" your chest and reverse the slump. You'll also find it easier to lift objects overhead, as well as perform overhead movements in sports.

WORKOUT GUIDELINES

Hold stretch for 30 seconds. Repeat 3 times. For a deeper stretch, hold a ½- or 1-pound weight in each hand.

EXPERT ADVICE

"Allow the heaviness of your arms to take you into a deep stretch," says Karen Clippinger, M.S.P.E., a Los Angeles based kinesiologist and instructor at UCLA. "The more you can relax and breathe in this position, the more you will feel open in the front of your shoulders and chest when you're through."

This reach can open your shoulder muscles even more thoroughly than a traditional shoulder stretch.

MISTAKES TO AVOID

➤ **Don't** arch your back; this strains your back muscles and spine.
➤ **Don't** walk your feet so far forward that you lose control of your position. You may slip or become unable to use your abdominals to maintain alignment.
➤ **Don't** throw your rib cage out or jut your chin to the ceiling, which can jam your shoulders up into your ears, and places stress on your neck and upper back muscles.

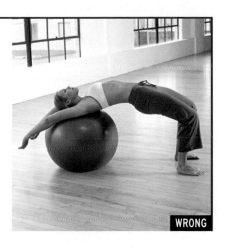

WRONG

This stretch can make a difference from your arms all the way down your spine.

THE RIGHT WAY

➤ Kneeling on a soft surface in front of a table or other sturdy support, raise your arms overhead, elbows straight and hands slightly wider than shoulder-width apart. Bend forward if necessary from hips until your palms rest on top of the support.

➤ Keeping torso straight, press your upper chest and head through your arms and down toward the floor until you feel a moderate stretch, but no pain, in the upper arms and shoulders as well as the muscles running down the sides of your back.

➤ Firmly contract your abs and pull your lower ribs in and down toward your pelvis.

➤ Stretch slowly; focus on relaxing your shoulder area.

MUSCLES STRETCHED
latissimus dorsi, anterior deltoid

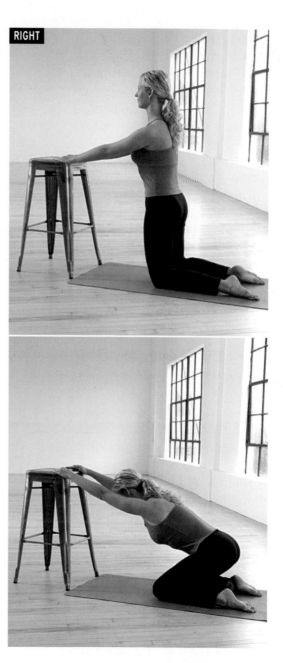

RIGHT

OVERHEAD LATS STRETCH

THE PAYOFF

Ever feel tight in the shoulders when reaching up to pull something off a high shelf or serving a tennis ball? Stiffness may be caused by tight latissimus dorsi muscles. This stretch helps relieve the tightness in your shoulders by stretching your lats. Neglecting to loosen up your lats may affect more than your ability to raise your arms overhead. It also makes you more likely to hunch over or roll your shoulders.

WORKOUT GUIDELINES

Repeat this stretch 2 to 3 times, feeling the muscles in your front shoulder region lengthen. To progress, sit deeper into the stretch.

EXPERT ADVICE

"Focus on stabilizing your torso by firmly contracting your abdominals and pulling your lower ribs in and down toward your pelvis," says Karen Clippinger, M.S.P.E., a Los Angeles-based kinesiologist and instructor at UCLA. "If you arch your back, the lat muscles will slack and you won't feel the sides of your torso stretching."

Neglecting to loosen up your lats makes you more likely to hunch over or roll your shoulders.

MISTAKES TO AVOID

➤ **Don't** round your spine or drop your head, which doesn't allow the lat muscles to stretch effectively.

➤ **Don't** place your arms too close together or hunch your shoulders up toward your ears; you won't get a sufficient stretch to the front shoulder region.

➤ **Don't** let your belly sag; you need to maintain a strong abdominal and lower back connection to stabilize your torso.

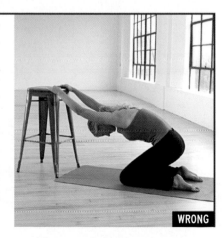

WRONG

Stretch and tone your body while calming your mind.

stretching

THE RIGHT WAY

➤ Kneel on all fours with your hands a few inches in front of your shoulders, fingers facing forward, knees directly under your hips, feet hip-width apart and toes turned under.

➤ Slowly lift your knees, keeping them bent, and press your hands into the floor. Extend spine and move your hips backward until your body forms a straight line from wrists to pelvis.

➤ Keeping spine elongated, straighten your legs, pressing your thighs back as you reach your heels toward the floor. (It's OK if they don't touch.) Your body should form a triangle with arms and legs straight. (If your hamstrings are tight, keep legs bent.)

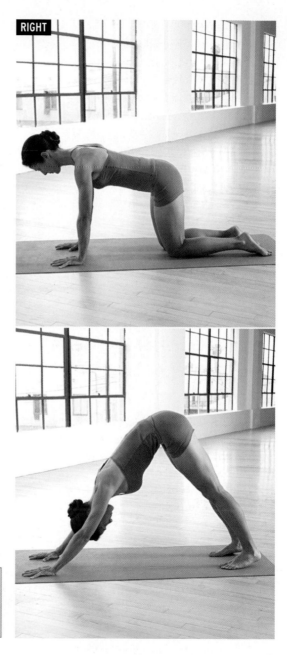

RIGHT

MUSCLES STRETCHED
erector spinae, hamstrings group, gastrocnemius, latissimus dorsi, anterior deltoid, posterior deltoid, pectoralis major, biceps, abdominals

DOWNWARD FACING DOG

THE PAYOFF

One of the fundamental yoga postures, this inverted pose provides an excellent stretch for your spine, shoulders, hamstrings and calf muscles. It also challenges your arms and legs to hold you up, toning the quadriceps, triceps and front shoulder muscles. You'll improve your balance, too.

WORKOUT GUIDELINES

Inhale as you lift your body, exhale as you straighten your legs. Breathe naturally as you hold, and focus on broadening your shoulders. If you're a beginner, hold the pose for 10-30 seconds. Do 3-5 reps, resting between each. Progress by holding the pose for at least a minute or more.

EXPERT ADVICE

"Instead of just holding this pose, really try to explore it," says Rodney Yee, co-director of the Piedmont Yoga studio in Oakland, Calif., and creator of Living Arts yoga videos. "Ask yourself: Which hand is supporting more weight? Which foot? Where does my spine feel long, and where does it feel jammed? Try to work your entire body evenly."

This inverted pose provides an excellent stretch for your spine, shoulders, hamstrings and calf muscles.

MISTAKES TO AVOID

➤ **Don't** arch your back or throw out your rib cage; you'll misalign the spine and place stress on your back and shoulder muscles.

➤ **Don't** try to press your heels down to touch the floor if you're inflexible. This could result in a torn calf or hamstring muscle.

➤ **Don't** hunch your shoulders up toward your ears rather than elongating your spine; you'll add stress to the upper-back and neck muscles.

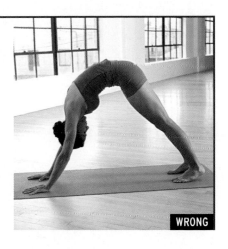

WRONG

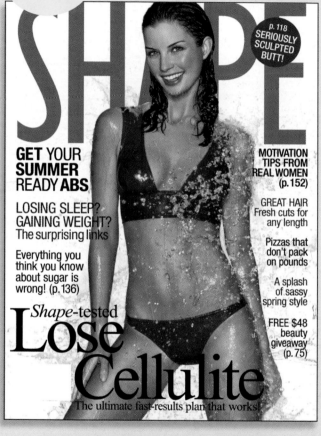